ck

AF843351

10 382 054 01

ON BSS

Management of Arterial Hyper

WITHDRAWN

THE AUTHORS

† **F. Gross,** Professor of Pharmacology, University of Heidelberg, Federal Republic of Germany

Z. Pisa, Head, Research Department of Preventive Cardiology, Institute for Clinical and Experimental Medicine (IKEM), Prague, Czechoslovakia (formerly, Chief Medical Officer, Cardiovascular Diseases, World Health Organization, Geneva, Switzerland)

T. Strasser, Secretary-General, World Hypertension League, Geneva, Switzerland (formerly, Medical Officer, Cardiovascular Diseases, World Health Organization, Geneva, Switzerland)

A. Zanchetti, Director, Institute of Clinical Medicine IV, University of Milan, Italy

A. Amery, Professor of Medicine, Department of Internal Medicine—Cardiology, University Hospital Gasthuisberg, Leuven, Belgium

C. W. G. Redman, Lecturer in Obstetric Medicine, Nuffield Department of Obstetrics and Gynaecology, John Radcliffe Hospital, Oxford, England

L. Wilhelmsen, Chief, Department of Medicine, Östra Hospital, University of Göteborg, Sweden

† Deceased 26 March 1984.

Management of Arterial Hypertension

A practical guide for the physician and allied health workers

by

F. Gross, Z. Pisa, T. Strasser and A. Zanchetti

with the assistance of:
A. Amery, C. Redman and L. Wilhelmsen

World
Health
Organization
Geneva 1984

NEWCASTLE UPON TYNE
POLYTECHNIC
LIBRARY
ACCESSION No. 1038205401
CLASS No. 616.132

ISBN 92 4 154197 0

© World Health Organization 1985

Publications of the World Health Organization enjoy copyright protection in accordance with the provisions of Protocol 2 of the Universal Copyright Convention. For rights of reproduction or translation of WHO publications, in part or *in toto*, application should be made to the Office of Publications, World Health Organization, Geneva, Switzerland. The World Health Organization welcomes such applications.

The designations employed and the presentation of the material in this publication do not imply the expression of any opinion whatsoever on the part of the Secretariat of the World Health Organization concerning the legal status of any country, territory, city or area or of its authorities, or concerning the delimitation of its frontiers or boundaries.

The mention of specific companies or of certain manufactures' products does not imply that they are endorsed or recommended by the World Health Organization in preference to others of a similar nature that are not mentioned. Errors and omissions excepted, the names of proprietary products are distinguished by initial capital letters.

The authors alone are responsible for the views expressed in this publication.

TYPESET IN INDIA
PRINTED IN ENGLAND
83/5964 – Macmillan/Spottiswoods 10,000

CONTENTS

Preface

Hypertension is a very common condition and is an important public health problem in all countries of the world—hence the World Health Organization's commitment to promote better control, management, and treatment. Although virtually symptomless, it is an important contributing cause to cerebrovascular, heart, and renal disease.

WHO's efforts in this field have included promoting the control of hypertension; analyses of, and recommendations for, the worldwide control of hypertension; special projects to demonstrate the feasibility of community control of hypertension; health care related research; and the production of health education material to help people understand the hazards of high blood pressure. The present volume is based on the report of a WHO Expert Committee on Arterial Hypertension[1] and is an attempt to provide practical and balanced information for all health workers on how to manage hypertensive patients.

Although the management of hypertension is a rapidly changing field, and new drugs are constantly being developed, they are not necessarily more useful than some older ones, and the *principles* of therapy will probably not change much in the course of a few years.

Practicality and clarity were the chief concerns of the authors in preparing the text and illustrations. Simplifications were both unavoidable and intentional.

[1] WHO Technical Report Series No. 628, 1978 (*Arterial hypertension*: report of a WHO Expert Committee).

Acknowledgements

The authors gratefully acknowledge the valuable contributions of Dr J. I. S. Robertson, MRC Blood Pressure Unit, Western Infirmary, Glasgow, Scotland, to the preparation of this book. The assistance of Dr G. P. Hodsman of the same Unit is also greatly appreciated.

1
INTRODUCTION

What is hypertension?

The term arterial hypertension describes the persistent elevation of (arterial) blood pressure. This definition is based on two critical features: *elevation* and *persistence*.

Elevated blood pressure values are a systolic pressure equal to or greater than 160 mmHg (21.3 kPa) and/or a diastolic pressure (5th phase) equal to or greater than 95 mmHg (127 kPa). Normal blood pressure in adults is equal to or below 140 mmHg (18.6 kPa) systolic and 90 mmHg (12.0 kPa) diastolic. The pressure values between elevated and normal are known as borderline (Fig. 1).

These limits apply to adults of both sexes of any age. The values for children that would be regarded as hypertensive are lower, but no precise figures have been generally accepted.

Persistent elevation of blood pressure can be ascertained only by repeated measurements over a longer period of observation. A single, casual finding of elevated blood pressure does not justify the diagnosis of hypertension (unless very high values are found). At least three blood pressure readings should be taken on each of at least two different occasions before declaring that a subject has hypertension (for more details see section 5).

Blood pressure varies during the day and is usually considerably lower at night. This applies to both normal and hypertensive subjects, but the latter still have higher values at night than normotensive individuals.

The arbitrary nature of diagnostic criteria

There is no natural dividing line between normal blood pressure and hypertension. The simplified definition proposed by WHO is based on

Fig. 1. Normal, borderline, and elevated blood pressure (mean values of 3 readings on 2 different occasions)

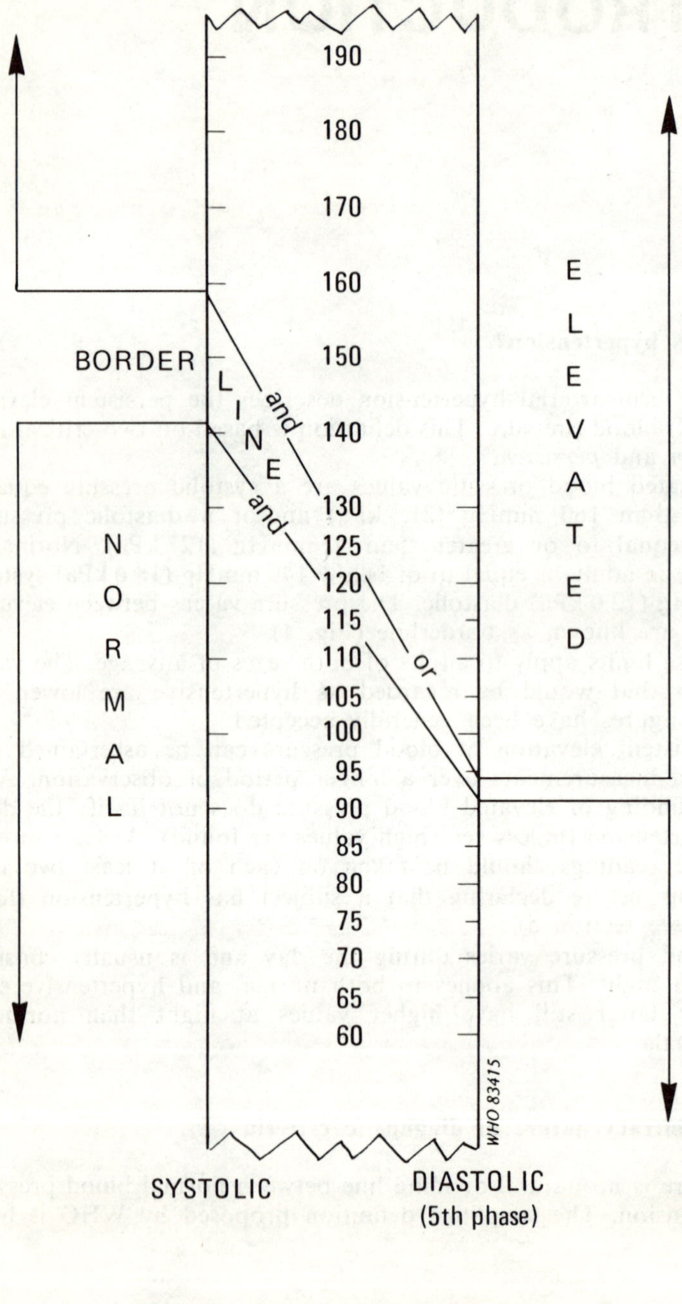

consensus. In any population, blood pressure values have a continuous, bell-shaped distribution skewed to the upper end (Fig. 2). Because of this it is not possible to distinguish clearly "pathological" from "normal" values.

Fig. 2. The continuous distribution of blood pressure values in a population

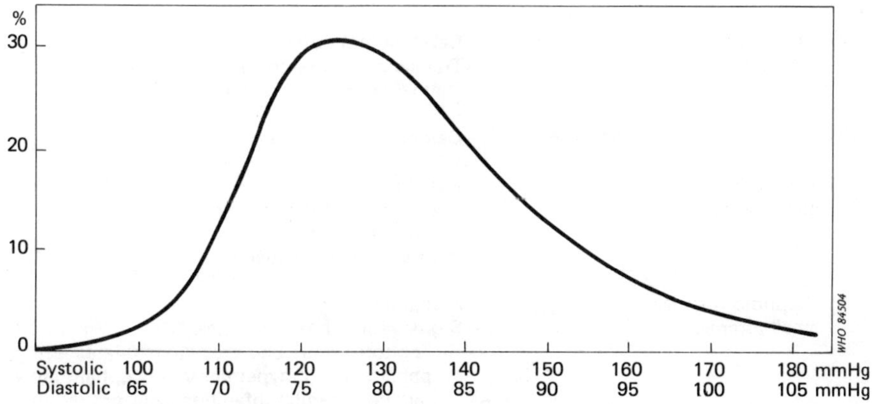

Blood pressure is a graded phenomenon, associated with graded risk. The higher the arterial pressure—systolic or diastolic—the greater the risk of complications and the shorter the life expectancy of the patient (see below). The discrete categories of "hypertensive" and "normal" levels of blood pressure are useful, practical simplifications, but it should always be remembered that blood pressure is a *quantitative* entity.

The diagnosis of hypertension alone does not necessarily indicate the need for drug treatment. Guidelines for management and treatment are given in sections 6–10.

The hazards of hypertension

Persistently elevated blood pressure imposes an increased workload on the heart, resulting eventually in left ventricular hypertrophy. If it is untreated, chronic marked hypertension may eventually lead to *hypertensive heart disease* which is a severe and potentially fatal condition involving dilatation and failure of the left ventricle. However, the signs of left ventricular hypertrophy may disappear after persistent and adequate therapy of moderate hypertension.

The changes in the arterial wall induced by chronic hypertension, and the clinical consequences, are summarized in Table 1.

The *malignant* (*accelerated*) *phase* is the most serious of all the complications of hypertension. Fortunately, it is uncommon. If

Table 1. Changes in the arterial walls provoked or promoted by high blood pressure, and the resulting clinical consequences

Changes in arterial wall	Clinical complications
(1) Atheroma	– Coronary heart disease – Cerebral thrombosis and infarction – Dissecting aneurysm
(2) Thromboembolism from atheroma	– Cerebral infarction – Transient cerebral ischaemic attacks – Retinal arterial occlusion
(3) Charcot-Bouchard aneurysms	– Cerebral haemorrhage
(4) Fatty hyalinosis and elastosis of small arterioles	– Renal impairment – Retinal arterial thickening and irregularity – Retinal arterial occlusion
(5) Fibrinoid necrosis of small arteries	– Malignant (accelerated) phase – Signs: retinal haemorrhages, "cotton-wool" and discrete exudates and papilloedema; hypertensive encephalopathy; renal glomerular infarction with proteinuria, haematuria and renal failure; cerebral haemorrhage

untreated, the malignant phase is fatal within a few months. The course of this phase may be abruptly terminated by a catastrophic cerebral haemorrhage or by cardiac failure; the patient who escapes or survives these events eventually succumbs to renal failure.

Hypertensive encephalopathy is a rare manifestation of severe hypertension. The cerebral arterioles are forcibly dilated by the very high arterial pressure and hence the brain is over-perfused, rapidly becoming oedematous. The symptoms are headache, with impairment of consciousness ranging from drowsiness and confusion to coma. Epileptiform fits occur in the later stages. The patient rapidly succumbs if the blood pressure is not promptly reduced. Hypertension is a more dominant risk factor in relation to stroke than it is for coronary heart disease, where it is one of several important risk factors.

Stroke (cerebral infarction and haemorrhage) and *coronary heart disease* (angina pectoris and especially myocardial infarction) are by far the most common complications of hypertension. Both conditions are the result of a number of influences, but hypertension is one of the principal pathogenic factors; its role as a risk factor has been assessed quantitatively in prospective epidemiological studies.

The probability that hypertensive subjects may develop the above conditions can be expressed in terms of absolute[1] and as relative risk.[2] The absolute risk of both stroke and myocardial infarction differs in various populations, in men and women, and at various ages; on the other hand, the relative risk due to high blood pressure seems to be rather uniform. Fig. 3 and 4 show the relative risks of stroke and myocardial infarction at various blood pressure levels.

With higher blood pressure values the risk increases more steeply, but subjects with only slightly raised blood pressure are already at a higher risk than those with normal or low values. Since in many populations there are many more individuals with slightly raised blood pressure than with severe hypertension, the resulting community attributable risk[3] of mild hypertension is greater than that of severe hypertension—although, clearly, the individual with severe hypertension is personally at a much greater risk (Fig. 5).

Fig. 3. Relative risk of developing stroke within 8 years in a 55-year old male related to systolic blood pressure levels

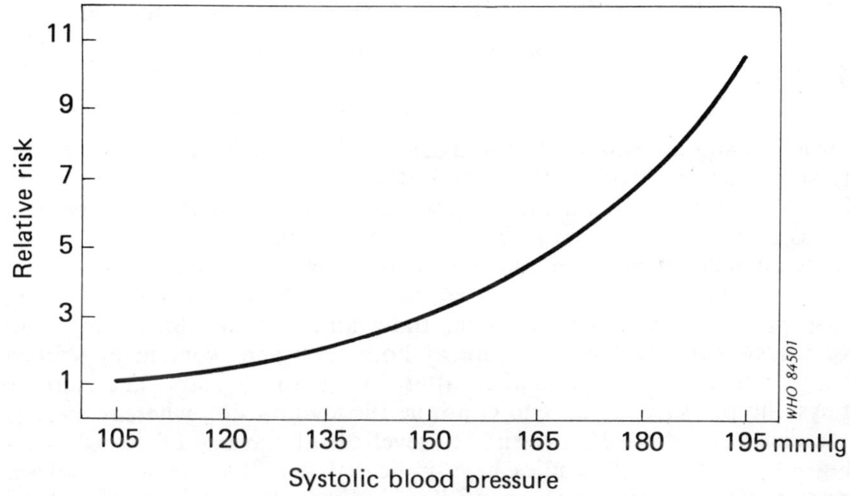

Hypertension around the world

The blood pressure ranges of a large proportion of the adult population in many parts of the world are associated with excess

---

[1] Absolute risk: the probability that a person will develop a disease within a defined period of time.

[2] Relative risk: a measure of the risk for a subject exposed to a given risk factor, compared with the risk for a non-exposed subject.

[3] Community attributable risk: portion of the expected incidence of a disease attributable to the prevalence or level of a risk factor in a defined population or community.

Fig. 4. Relative risk of developing myocardial infarction within 5 years in a 45-year old male related to systolic blood pressure levels

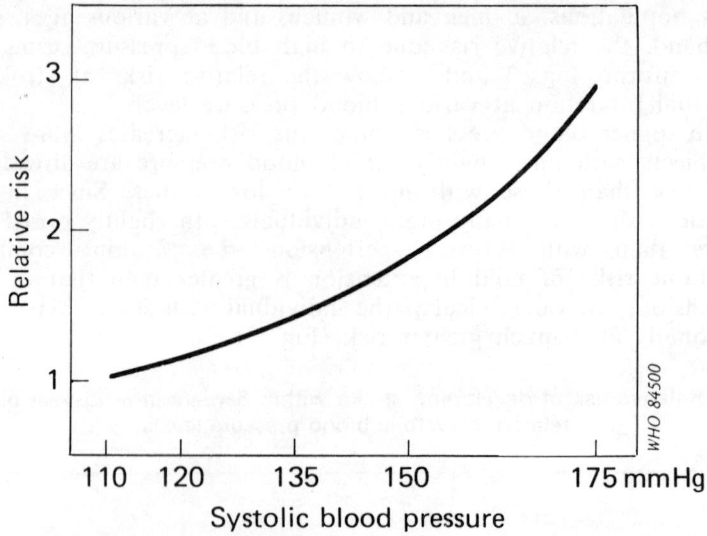

morbidity and mortality. From 5–18% of adults have casual[1] blood pressure above 160 mmHg (21.3 kPa) systolic and/or 95 mmHg (12.7 kPa) diastolic. Data on the prevalence of hypertension, as defined in this manual, are not available; nevertheless, findings based on casual measurements do have definite epidemiological importance.

Virtually all surveys in developed and developing countries, including those from Africa, Latin America, India and Oceania, have shown an age-related rise in blood pressure in both men and women; in women this phenomenon is more marked after the age of 50 years. The increase in systolic pressure appears to continue throughout life, whereas there is a tendency for diastolic pressure to level off at the age of 55–60 years (Fig. 6). Longitudinal studies have indicated that the increase in blood pressure with age is more marked in individuals in whom the blood pressure initially recorded at any age was higher than normal. In young adults in the United States of America, the increase in pressure with age is greater in blacks than in whites; hence, there is a significant excess prevalence of high blood pressure in the black population. However, there are certain notable exceptions. In some small, mostly isolated communities in which generally low blood pressure values are found

[1] Casual blood pressure: values obtained on *ad hoc* examination.

Fig. 5. Some quantitative relationships in hypertension care: a conceptual scheme

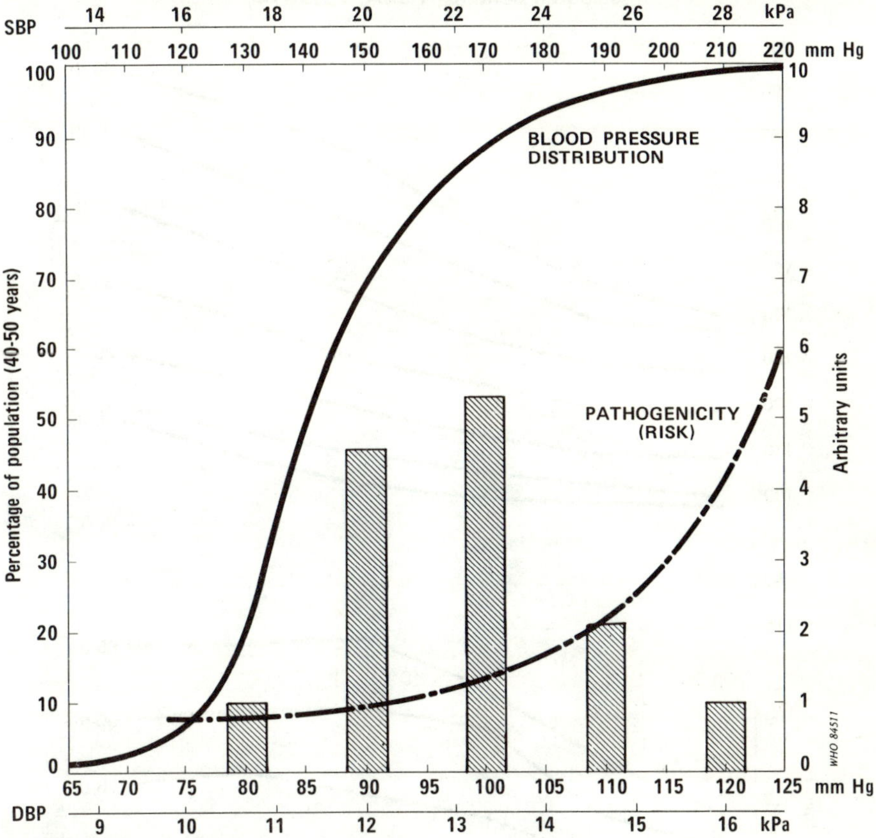

The bars illustrate the community attributable risk of hypertension.

The blood pressure distribution curve has been idealized in order to accommodate both systolic and diastolic pressures on a single curve.

there is no observed increase with age. The importance of such exceptions is discussed in section 4.

Geographical aspects

People living in the mountainous regions of South America tend to have low blood pressure; however, these levels increase and also show a normal rise with age when the high-altitude residents migrate to the less primitive lowland regions. Interestingly, in Ethiopia, where highlanders have a higher socioeconomic status than lowlanders, they also have

Fig. 6. Systolic and diastolic blood pressure levels of adults aged 18–74 years, by selected centiles[a] (USA, 1971–74)

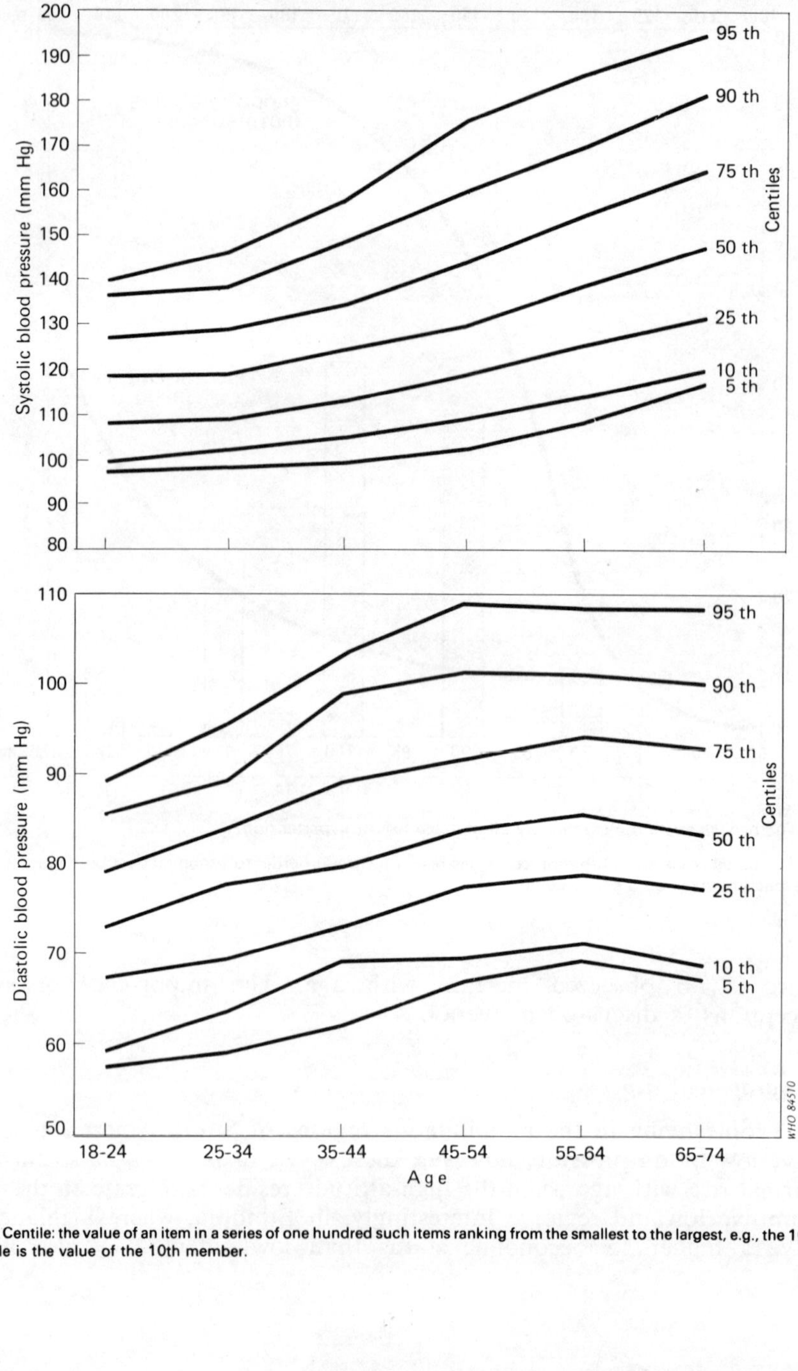

[a] Centile: the value of an item in a series of one hundred such items ranking from the smallest to the largest, e.g., the 10th centile is the value of the 10th member.

higher average blood pressures. Both Tokelauans migrating to New Zealand and Easter Islanders migrating to Chile show a subsequent rise in blood pressure. Some small communities have a tendency to higher than average blood pressures; for instance on the Hebridean island of Tiree higher pressures have been observed than on the mainland of west Scotland.

Although many of these studies are interesting, they fail to disentangle the complicated and sometimes conflicting influences of genetics, geographical location, culture, socioeconomic status, and diet.

2
HOW TO MEASURE BLOOD PRESSURE

IT is important not to be misled by the apparent simplicity of the procedure for measuring blood pressure. However, valid results can be obtained by observing basic rules concerning the patient, the instrument, the examiner himself, and the environment.

The patient

Most spurious diagnoses of hypertension are probably due to quick measurements made on unprepared and tense patients.[1] Before starting the measurement, the person to be examined should have been seated for at least 5 minutes, relaxing in a comfortable chair in a pleasant and reassuring atmosphere and must not have made any vigorous effort during the preceding 30 minutes, smoked, or taken coffee. The patient's upper arm should have been previously stripped and should be placed on a soft arm rest.

Measurement of arterial pressure with the patient in the sitting position is the most practical method. Measurement of arterial pressure with the patient in the lying position and again after he has been standing for 1–5 minutes may give useful clinical information about the hypertensive patient, particularly when under treatment.

It is also valuable to record the heart rate at the same time as the blood pressure measurement; this is particularly important during treatment with certain drugs (e.g., vasodilators, adrenergic inhibitors, and beta-adrenoceptor blockers).

[1] In the present context, "patient" includes healthy individuals undergoing a health check.

Fig. 7. Commonest faults found in sphygmomanometers

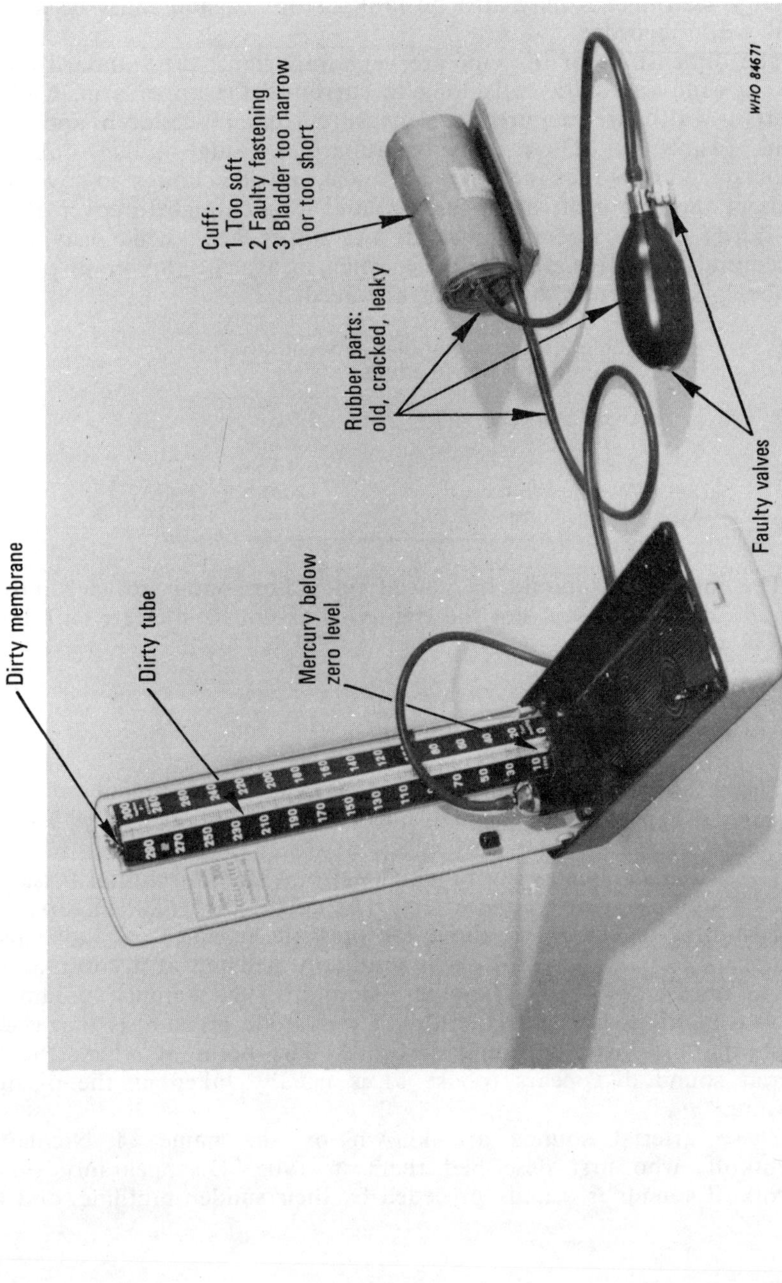

The instrument

Mercury sphygmomanometers are recommended since they are more reliable than the aneroid-type instruments (i.e., with a pointer). However, mercury instruments may also be faulty (Fig. 7), and must be kept in good working order.

The dimensions of the cuff are very important; the standard cuff is 12.5 cm wide and sufficiently long to surround the upper arm. Cuffs of different width are required for measurements in children and obese adults (Table 2). These dimensions are a rough guide only; the important point is that the inner bag must be wide enough to cover two-thirds of the length of the upper arm and long enough to cover at least two-thirds of the circumference of the upper arm, while leaving the antecubital fossa free. For instance, when measuring the blood pressure of obese adults, cuffs 40 cm long are needed.

Table 2. Recommended cuff-width for children and obese adults

Under one year	2.5 cm
1–3 years	5–6 cm
4–8 years	9–10 cm
Average adults	12.5 cm
Obese adults	14 cm

The instrument should be placed on a horizontal surface, and the cuff adjusted firmly, but not too tightly so as not to interfere with blood flow in the arm.

The examiner

The examiner should be trained in the measurement of blood pressure. If appropriately trained, nurses are as good at it as physicians, and often they are better.

The examiner locates the brachial pulse in the antecubital fossa and places a stethoscope over the artery. The cuff is then inflated rapidly to 20–30 mmHg (2.7–4.0 kPa) above the pressure at which the radial pulse disappears to palpation, then it is gradually deflated at a constant rate of 2–3 mmHg (0.27–0.4 kPa) per second. The mercury column is watched continuously and carefully. The systolic pressure is that one at which the first arterial sound is heard. The point at which the last arterial sound disappears (phase 5) is usually taken as the diastolic pressure.

These arterial sounds are known by the name of Nicolai S. Korotkoff, who first described them in 1905. Disappearance of the Korotkoff sounds is usually preceded by their sudden muffling, and this is known as phase 4. Some physicians prefer phase 4 disappearance as the indicator of diastolic pressure.

The readings are made at the closest two-millimetre mark on the scale. After having taken the first blood pressure readings, the examiner completely deflates the cuff and then proceeds in the same way to obtain two further readings.

The environment

As mentioned above, blood pressure measurement should take place in a pleasant and reassuring atmosphere. Room temperature should be around 21°C, since low environmental temperature causes an elevation of blood pressure and excessive heat provokes tachycardia. The room should be quiet to ensure reliable ausculation of the arterial sounds.

In the presence of cardiac arrhythmias (e.g., atrial fibrillation), repeated measurements are needed in order to obtain a satisfactory approximation of the average systolic and diastolic pressures.

When examining children, it is important to obtain their confidence and to ensure a quiet environment. The phase 4 sound often gives a better indication of diastolic pressure in children, because the arterial sound may persist until the cuff pressure has fallen to zero. In pregnant women, the phase 4 sound is also used for the determination of diastolic pressure.

Other devices for blood pressure measurement

Aneroid sphygmomanometers are subject to inaccuracies and should be regularly checked against a mercury column, either with both devices attached directly to the cuff or by using a Y-tube. Several methods have been used to simplify the signal received, the Korotkoff sound having been transformed into visual signals, digital displays, or transcribed from the recording device. Some machines have been adapted for long-term, semi-automatic recording of blood pressure levels at pre-set intervals over several hours. All these devices should be rigorously and repeatedly tested against the standard method. In infants under 2 years of age, one of the instruments using the Doppler principle is recommended.

Self-measurement of blood pressure

After suitable but simple training, a subject can measure his or her own blood pressure. Inexpensive devices are widely available commercially, including automatic devices and mercury or aneroid sphygmomanometers with a stethoscope head incorporated into the cuff. Self-measurement can take place at home, in pharmacies, or department stores, mostly with automatic devices. While measurements in public places should be discouraged, self-measurements at home are most often taken in a relaxed state, under optimal environmental conditions, and it is notable that in these circumstances individuals often report lower arterial pressure values than those obtained by a doctor or a nurse during periodical examinations. Home self-measurement provides more data that can be used by the physician in deciding whether and how to treat, and may also improve the patients' compliance and cooperation. However, patients should always report the results of self-measurement to their physicians, and unsupervised self-medication or medication on the advice of pharmacists should be actively discouraged. Both the ability of the patient to measure his own blood pressure and the reliability of the equipment used should be periodically checked.

3 DETECTING HYPERTENSION

HYPERTENSION is usually symptomless. Symptoms ascribed by patients to hypertension, such as headache, fatigue, dizziness or drumming in the ears, are only rarely due to hypertension.

The popular belief that these symptoms are indicative of hypertension may have contributed to the fact that until recently only about half the number of hypertensive individuals were aware of their disease. The second, and perhaps more important, cause of under-diagnosis by the medical profession has been insufficient awareness of the pathogenic and prognostic importance of moderate and mild hypertension.

Since hypertension is a symptomless disease, its *detection is the responsibility of the doctor*. Unless doctors search for hypertension regularly, many cases will remain undiagnosed or will be diagnosed late (see section 11).

There are several ways of detecting hypertension and these are presented in Table 3.

Systematic screening is usually carried out as a special project. The project may be organized specifically to measure blood pressure, or

Table 3. Possible methods of detecting hypertension

Systematic screening programme
- For hypertension only
- Health surveys
  - community-wide
  - occupational groups
  - house-to-house surveys

Casual screening
- Self-screening
- Health examinations (including occupational medicine)
- Incidental screening

blood pressure measurement may be carried out in association with another screening programme, such as fluorography, that includes an entire population or specific population groups.

Another way of detecting hypertension is by means of health surveys of populations or population samples. Such surveys, usually carried out for research purposes, should include blood pressure measurement in addition to a number of other examinations.

Screening programmes may be applied to the entire population of a community, to selected occupational groups (e.g., bank employees, policemen, factory workers), or to households (house-to-house screening).

Screening programmes for hypertension may be carried out easily and at relatively low cost. However, their effectiveness has been shown to be quite low since only a fraction of those requiring treatment seek further medical assistance and start regular therapy. Conversely, a large proportion of individuals found to have elevated blood pressure when measured under unstandardized conditions, are eventually found to be "normal" when followed up. Nevertheless, screening programmes, including casual self-screening with automatic devices in public places and pharmacies, are useful in promoting public awareness of hypertension as a health problem.

It is obvious that any health examination should include the measurement of blood pressure, whether it is being done in the context of occupational medicine (periodic health examinations of workers and employees) or for other reasons, e.g., for obtaining a driver's licence, or in recruits. In addition, the blood pressure should be measured in any subject who consults the medical or health services for any reason. This way of searching for hypertension is known as *incidental screening* and should be the most effective way of detecting hypertension since in any population a considerable proportion of the people see a physician or have some contact with the health services at least once a year.

It should be remembered, however, that a casual blood pressure measurement cannot be used to diagnose hypertension. Elevated blood pressure found on casual measurement indicates to the subject and the physician that full measurement of the blood pressure should be performed, as described in section 2.

Incidental screening may raise some ethical problems. It has been pointed out that the physician may not have the right to diagnose hypertension in a patient who comes to see him for a defined, minor, and completely unrelated ailment such as coryza, dandruff, or an ingrown toe-nail. As for many other ethical controversies, no absolute norms can be established. The physician should briefly and politely ask for the patient's consent to take his blood pressure. If the patients are adequately cared for when found to have elevated blood pressure, the great majority will probably appreciate rather than resent the physician's additional effort in making the measurement.

In summary, the solution to the community-wide detection of hypertension lies in making blood pressure measurement part of every health check including all outpatient and health examinations, in the sick and healthy, and at any age, including childhood. Any patient found to have high blood pressure should be followed up and treated, if subsequently found to require therapy.

4 WHAT CAUSES HYPERTENSION?

IN 96–99% of cases of hypertension, the cause or causes of blood pressure elevation will not be clearly identifiable (*essential or primary hypertension*). Nevertheless, it is important to recognize the cause whenever possible because its removal may obviate the need for treatment with antihypertensive drugs. In some cases, the cause can be removed easily, once it has been recognized; in other cases the responsible lesions may require medical or surgical attention, quite apart from the raised blood pressure. Hypertension with an identifiable cause is known as *secondary hypertension* (see Table 4 for a list of the possible causes).

Table 4. Causes of secondary hypertension

(1) Hypertension due to the administration of drugs and chemicals
- hormonal contraceptives (containing estrogen)
- non-steroidal antirheumatic agents such as indometacin
- corticosteroids and corticotrophin (ACTH)
- liquorice and carbenoxolone
- others

(2) Hypertensive disease of pregnancy

(3) Organic diseases
- coarctation of the aorta
- renal diseases (renal artery stenosis; glomerulonephritis; pyelonephritis; radiation nephritis; renal tuberculosis; renal cysts; hydronephrosis; renal tumours, including renin-secreting tumours; renal failure)
- diseases of the adrenal cortex (primary hyperaldosteronism; Cushing's syndrome; tumours producing excess of other corticosteroids, e.g., corticosterone and desoxycortone; inborn errors of corticosteroid biosynthesis)
- diseases of the adrenal medula (phaeochromocytoma)

Essential (primary) hypertension

This is defined as hypertension for which there is no identifiable cause. Obviously, unlike certain forms of secondary hypertension, only symptomatic treatment is possible.

The tendency to develop essential hypertension is inherited, probably in a polygenic fashion.[1] However, in addition, a number of environmental factors play an important role by contributing to the full expression of hypertension, and these are of predominant concern in exploring the possibilities of prevention and non-drug treatment of hypertension, since obviously, nothing can be done to influence the genetic element.

Certain communities with a generally low level of blood pressure have excited considerable interest because if the factor or factors responsible for the maintenance of low blood pressure could be identified, this would have important implications for prevention and treatment. Such communities are widely scattered geographically, being found on various Pacific islands, in both mountainous and jungle areas of South America, as well as at a variety of locations in Africa and Asia. Despite the ethnic diversity, these communities share common features. They are small and isolated. A high level of physical activity is combined with a low average energy intake, often with periods when the food supply is clearly deficient. Salt intake is usually low, almost invariably being less than 4 g daily and often substantially less. Potassium intake is usually high. Members of the community are closely interdependent. One or several of these factors combined might be of importance in determining the low level of blood pressure. The importance of environmental, rather than genetic, factors in determining low blood pressure in these communities is underlined by the observation that people migrating from such areas to more complex societies generally show the usual rise in blood pressure with age. Such migration involves the modification of several environmental factors simultaneously; hence, it is not easy to disentangle their respective influences. The following aspects nevertheless appear likely to be important:

(1) *Body weight.* There is a close relationship between blood pressure and weight. This applies to both children and adults, and has been found in developing as well as in technically-developed societies. Individuals who gain more weight with advancing years show a more rapid rise in arterial pressure. Weight reduction has been seen to be accompanied by a fall in arterial pressure.

(2) *Sodium intake.* A very high intake of sodium chloride (more than 14 g/day) will cause a detectable increase, while a very low intake (less

[1] Polygenic inheritance: heredity due to the action of many genes.

than 1 g/day) reduces arterial pressure. The influence of a modest reduction in dietary sodium chloride, from around 5 g to 2.5 g/day, is still controversial. The restriction of intake of sodium potentially offers one of the most ready means of primary prevention of high blood pressure and is perhaps the best non-drug treatment. The role, if any, of potassium in the pathogenesis of hypertension is not yet clear.

(3) *Alcohol.* An association between a high intake of ethyl alcohol and high blood pressure has been reported in a number of studies, but the mechanism of the association remains unclear.

(4) *Psychosocial factors.* The role of psychosocial factors in the pathogenesis of hypertension has aroused considerable interest. There is little evidence that harm can result from short-term blood pressure increases in response to acute psychological stimuli. On the other hand, there are reports that factory workers subjected continually to intensive noise have higher mean blood pressures than others working in quieter surroundings in the same factory. Studies on migrant populations indicate that long-term exposure to adverse psychosocial circumstances might lead to hypertension.

(5) *Exercise.* Although a number of studies have reported on the effects of physical training, as yet no clearcut changes in blood pressure have been demonstrated.

(6) *Smoking.* No causal relationship exists between smoking and hypertension, but smoking is an additional cardiovascular risk factor to the patient. Smoking combined with the consumption of coffee has a short-term pressor effect.

Secondary hypertension[1]

Drugs and chemicals

Hypertension caused by the ingestion of drugs and chemicals is by far the most important form of secondary hypertension for several reasons: often, it is of iatrogenic origin; usually, the elevated blood pressure values revert to normal when the causal substance is no longer ingested; and, in principle, this type of hypertension can be easily prevented.

Estrogen–progestogen oral contraceptives rank first among the drugs with the potential to cause hypertension. In women taking 30 μg or more of estrogen daily, blood pressure rises almost invariably for up to 2 years and then remains at the same level for as long as the subject continues to take this type of contraceptive. In nearly all cases, blood pressure reverts to pre-treatment levels within 3 months of withdrawal of the contraceptive. The magnitude of the rise in pressure varies individually:

[1] See also section 10.

the mean rise is about 15 mmHg (2.0 kPa) systolic and 7–10 mmHg (0.9–1.3 kPa) diastolic. In some individuals marked elevations can occur, and occasionally patients have been found to be in the malignant phase of hypertension. Progestogen taken alone does not result in elevation of the blood pressure.

The importance of oral contraceptives in raising blood pressure can not be over-emphasized. Oral contraceptives should not be taken unless the blood pressure is normal, and it should be checked at least twice a year. If the blood pressure is found to rise during an oral contraceptive regimen, a change should be made to an alternative method of contraception. It is clearly both illogical and wrong to administer antihypertensive drugs while the patient continues to take a pressor drug.

Liquorice is frequently eaten in sweets and is also used occasionally as a treatment for peptic ulcer. It contains glycyrrhizinic acid, which has a mineralocorticoid effect. Thus, persons who consume large quantities of liquorice may develop raised blood pressure accompanied by sodium retention and potassium depletion. The drug carbenoxolone contains the same active ingredient as liquorice and thus may have a similar action. The biochemical abnormalities and associated hypertension accompanying the ingestion of liquorice or carbenoxolone resolve following withdrawal of these substances.

The administration of corticosteroids or corticotrophin (ACTH) may increase the arterial pressure. With corticotrophin it seems probable that this blood pressure increase is mainly as a result of adrenal release of corticotrophin-sensitive mineralocorticoids, although other classes of corticosteroid may be involved.

Non-steroidal anti-inflammatory agents, such as indometacin, may result in blood pressure elevation.

A transitory rise in pressure may follow the abuse of nasal decongestants, such as phenylpropanolamine and other catecholamines, such as ephedrine hydrochloride or amphetamine. Certain appetite-reducing drugs may have similar effects.

The ingestion of food and drink containing large amounts of tyramine (certain cheeses, beers, wines, pickled herring, and chicken livers) can precipitate dangerous bouts of raised blood pressure in patients taking mono-amine oxidase inhibitors, such as pargyline.

Coarctation of the aorta

This congenital abnormality is characterized by a narrowing of the aorta, usually adjacent to the insertion of the ductus arteriosus. It gives rise to a characteristic form of hypertension in which the femoral pulses are diminished or absent and delayed in comparison with the radial pulses. Usually an extensive collateral circulation develops around the thorax. Surgical correction is the appropriate treatment.

Renal disease

A wide variety of renal and renal arterial diseases can cause or aggravate hypertension. These include renal artery stenosis; a variety of parenchymal renal lesions typically affecting both kidneys and in which distinct impairment of renal function usually accompanies hypertension (acute and chronic glomerulonephritis, nephropathy due to the abuse of analgesics, polycystic disease, chronic pyelonephritis); and some unilateral renal lesions (hydronephrosis, cyst, various benign and malignant tumours, unilateral tuberculosis).

End-stage renal failure resulting from bilateral renal disease requires regular dialysis; usually blood pressure control is achieved or at least greatly facilitated by this procedure. When a unilateral renal lesion is found in a hypertensive patient, removal of the affected kidney may sometimes lower the blood pressure, although this does not always occur. Nevertheless, certain of these lesions require nephrectomy for reasons other than that of blood pressure control.

Other causes

Conditions such as Conn's syndrome (primary hyperaldosteronism), Cushing's syndrome, phaeochromocytoma, and intracranial tumours leading to hypertension, are, in general practice, quite rare. They are described in textbooks of medicine.

Fig. 8. Scheme of causal relationships leading to hypertension[a]

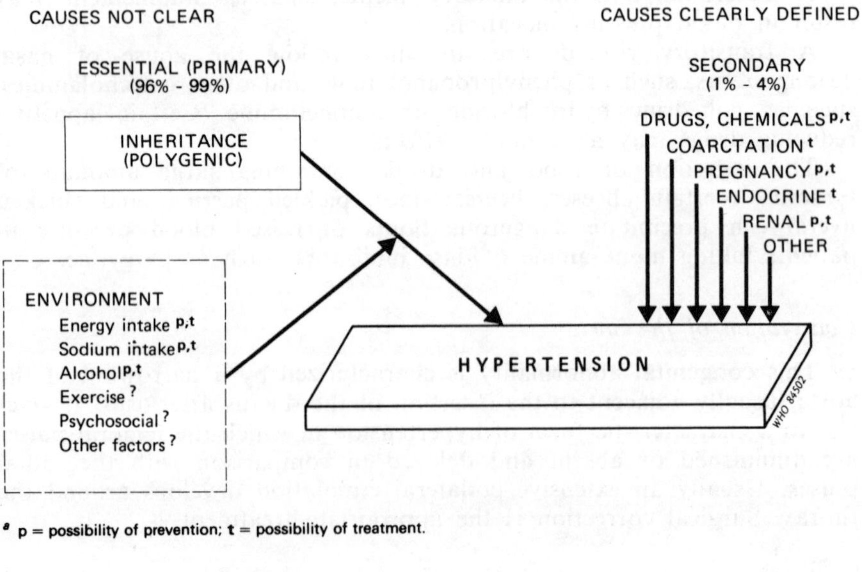

[a] p = possibility of prevention; t = possibility of treatment.

Summary of the causes of hypertension

The causal relationships leading to arterial hypertension are summarized in Fig. 8. Clearly defined causes are responsible for a small proportion of all cases of hypertension observed in general practice. (Hospital inpatients are highly selected and therefore are not representative of the population.) Elimination, withdrawal, or treatment of the clearly defined causes may often lead to the prevention or cure of hypertension. On the other hand, despite the fact that the relationships have not been established with sufficient clarity, intervention with respect to environmental factors probably involved in the expression of the genetic factors offers possibilities for the treatment (section 7) and perhaps prevention of essential hypertension. The mechanisms of the pathogenesis of hypertension are still poorly understood, including the question of how environmental factors influence the manifestation of genetic predispositions. This, however, does not rule out therapeutic or preventive action, when pragmatically justified.

5 ASSESSMENT OF THE HYPERTENSIVE PATIENT

AT first glance, the assessment of a hypertensive patient seems to be a simple task. In fact, the diagnostic process for hypertension is far from being a plain, uncomplicated procedure. However, major mistakes can be avoided by adhering to a few simple rules. The recommended sequence of action is given in Fig. 9.

The first task is to confirm or otherwise the existence of hypertension, defined as *chronic* blood pressure elevation (see Introduction). As mentioned above, it is inadmissible to start drug treatment—or even to initiate elaborate laboratory or other investigations—before the existence of hypertension is firmly established. No subject should be labelled as a hypertensive unless the values of at least 3 measurements taken on at least 2 separate occasions are in the hypertension range as shown in Fig. 1.

If this procedure is followed, the diagnosis will be confirmed only in some of those who were originally considered as potential hypertensives. Nevertheless, the persons in whom hypertension is not confirmed should be followed up after 6–12 months, unless it can be safely assumed that the first reading was erroneous or caused by some known external circumstance. The follow-up of individuals with occasional blood pressure elevation is needed because even single, casual elevated blood pressure values have a definite prognostic significance, and a number of such individuals may well develop a sustained blood pressure elevation at a later stage.

When hypertension has been confirmed, the physician must proceed as follows:

- inform the patient;
- assess the severity of the existing hypertension;
- assess the patient's overall cardiovascular risk;
- search for possible causes of the hypertension; and, if needed,
- carry out an extended examination to define and document the causes.

Fig. 9. Assessment of the hypertensive patient—sequence of action to be followed

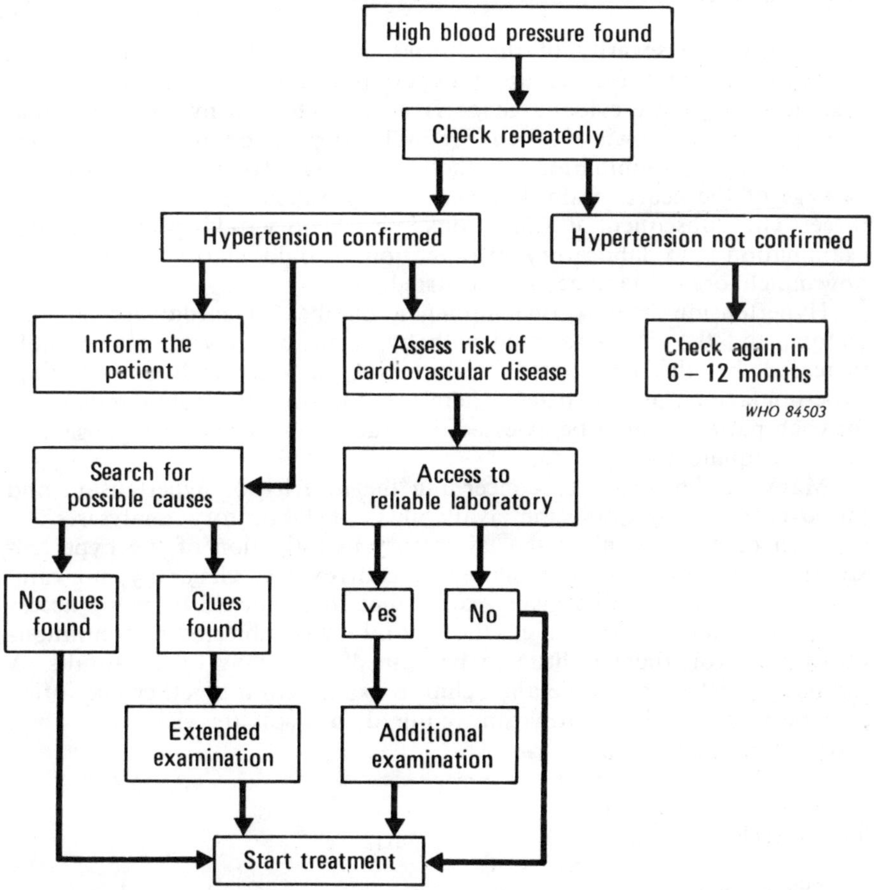

Informing the patient

It is indispensable to establish a good patient–doctor relationship at the very beginning for there to be satisfactory cooperation between the patient and the doctor, and for the patient to be adequately informed. Although this statement may apply to any disease, detailed information is of particular importance to hypertensive patients, because the disease is mostly symptomless and life-long. Proper explanations should be given to the patient for two reasons. Needless anxiety can be avoided, by explaining the benefits of treatment and the good prognosis of consistently treated hypertension; the patient should not, however, underestimate the risks of hypertension.

Assessment of the severity of the disease and the overall cardiovascular risk

Usually, the severity of the disease is assessed by classifying each case into one of three stages of hypertension. In stage I, no signs of organic changes are evident. Stage II is characterized by left ventricular hypertrophy, narrowing of the retinal arteries, or moderate kidney damage, or a combination of these. In stage III there is advanced damage of the heart, brain, kidney, or eyegrounds, or a combination of these. The subsequent examinations, i.e., history taking and physical examination and laboratory examination, should clarify whether and how much organ damage has occurred.

Hypertension is only one among a number of cardiovascular risk factors, and the risk associated with hypertension may be considerably increased by the presence of other risk factors, such as smoking, hyperlipidaemia, and diabetes. Therefore, the overall cardiovascular risk for each patient should be assessed, in order to establish a prognosis and begin adequate therapy.

Many of the questions concerning the severity of hypertension and the overall risk require the availability of laboratory analyses. The question of how extensive the laboratory investigation of the hypertensive patient should be is a matter of controversy. Generally, no valid recommendations can be given except that there should be ready access to a reliable laboratory. Unless the laboratory is subjected to continuous quality control, there is little to be gained by relying on its results. A well taken history and a detailed clinical examination together may often provide much of the information required to assess the risk factors and stages of hypertension.

The search for causes

The search for any potentially curable causes of blood pressure elevation, i.e., the diagnosis of secondary forms of hypertension, is a two-stage process. Although identifiable causes are uncommon, at least a limited search should always be made. This search should be more extensive in children and young adults than in older patients because in young people the proportion of cases with secondary forms of hypertension may be higher; also, they will have to tolerate the side-effects of hypotensive drugs for the longest time, if no remediable cause can be found.

During the first stage of this search, the examiner should seek information on the following subjects: use of oral contraceptives; ingestion of steroids or non-steroidal anti-inflammatory drugs; ingestion of liquorice: ingestion of carbenoxolone or analgesics; evidence of past or present renal disease, particularly urinary tract infection, trauma, and haematuria; signs and symptoms suggestive of phaeochromocytoma, including headache, pallor, anxiety, and attacks of sweating. During the clinical examination, attention should be paid to the palpation of the femoral pulses, since their absence may indicate coarctation of the aorta; the presence of Cushing's syndrome should be noted; further examinations include abdominal or loin murmurs, palpation of the kidneys, and inspection of the skin for neurofibromatosis.

If, after the above examinations and questions no apparent cause is found, the patient should be judged to have essential (primary) hypertension, and should be considered for treatment. However, if a clue to the cause of hypertension is found, the physician should refer the patient to a specialist or a hospital where an extensive examination can be undertaken to determine whether the patient's condition is, indeed, curable by surgical or other means.

Obviously, the search for possible causes, the assessment of the severity of hypertension and of the overall cardiovascular risk are elements of a single, coherent, and continuous diagnostic process that is carried out by the three classical methods of history taking, physical examination, and laboratory investigation. Tables 5–7 summarize the main items the physician should consider. The principal difficulty during diagnosis is to find the right measure for diagnostic work-up in a given situation. It is inadmissible to diagnose hypertension in a superficial way, since it is a lifelong disease and therapy may have serious implications for the patient. Also, the patient should not be exposed to a

Table 5. History

A. *Risk factors*
- Family history of hypertension and cardiovascular disease
- Family and personal history of hyperlipidaemia
- Family and personal history of diabetes mellitus
- Smoking habits
- Obesity; amount of physical exercise
- Personality of the patient; social environment

B. *Symptoms suggesting secondary hypertension*
- Family history of renal disease (polycystic kidney)
- Renal disease, urinary tract infection, haematuria, analgesic abuse (parenchymal renal disease)
- Oral contraceptives, liquorice, carbenoxolone, nasal drops (hypertension due to drugs)
- Episodes of sweating, headache, anxiety (phaeochromocytoma).
- Episodes of muscle weakness and tetany (hyperaldosteronism).

C. *Symptoms of organ damage*
- *Brain and eyes*: headache, vertigo, impaired vision, transient ischaemic attacks, sensory or motor deficit
- *Heart*: palpitations, chest pain, shortness of breath, ankle-swelling
- *Kidney*: thirst, polyuria, nocturia, haematuria
- *Peripheral arteries*: cold extremities, intermittent claudication

Table 6. Physical examination

Signs suggesting secondary hypertension
- Features of Cushing's syndrome
- Skin stigmata of neurofibromatosis (phaeochromocytoma)
- Palpation of enlarged kidneys (polycystic kidney)
- Ausculation of abdominal murmurs (renovascular hypertension)
- Auscultation of precordial or chest murmurs (aortic coarctation)
- Diminished and delayed femoral pulses and reduced leg blood pressure (aortic coarctation)

Signs of organ damage
- *Brain*: murmurs over neck arteries, motor or sensory defects
- *Retina*: fundoscopic examination
- *Heart*: location and characteristics of apical impulse, abnormal cardiac rhythms, ventricular gallop, pulmonary rales, dependent oedema
- *Peripheral arteries*: absence, reduction, or asymmetry of pulses, cold extremities, ischaemic skin lesions.

series of unjustified examinations. However, if therapeutic action is needed, it should not be withheld or even delayed because of lack of laboratory facilities. Sound judgement has to be applied.

Laboratory investigations

A detailed history and physical examination help to indicate the laboratory investigations needed; these tests will be rather simple in the majority of patients with mild or moderate hypertension and more detailed in severe or complicated hypertension. Full laboratory investigation may be neither necessary nor useful in certain patients. It may entail unnecessary discomfort and risk and may be excessively costly for the community or individual. Detailed evaluation with complex investigations should be reserved for patients with severe or resistant hypertension.

The minimum laboratory investigation needed is a matter of debate. However, it is agreed that investigations should progress from the most simple to the more complicated. It is always better to repeat simple tests for which the results are doubtful, rather than to perform a complex investigation at an early stage. The younger the patient, the higher the pressure, and the faster the development of hypertension, the more detailed the diagnostic examination should be, and the more assiduous the search for potentially curable causes of arterial hypertension.

Laboratory investigations are classified as follows and described in detail in the subsequent pages.

- *Strongly recommended tests*: to be performed on all hypertensive patients. These tests are simple and cheap yet provide basic information about renal and cardiac function.

- *Additional tests*: other simple tests that may be usefully performed when the facilities are available and additional information is desirable.
- *Extended evaluation*: performed by the hospital doctor or specialist for a more detailed study of complicated hypertension or to search for a curable cause of hypertension whenever the history, physical examination, or simpler tests suggest this possibility.

Strongly recommended tests

(*a*) *Urine analysis.* A dip-stick test for the presence of protein, sugar, or blood in the urine should be performed for all cases. If this is positive, laboratory verification is necessary, together with microscopic examination of the urinary sediment. This latter test should always be performed in a patient with suspected renal parenchymal disease.

(*b*) *Plasma creatinine concentration.* This gives information on renal (glomerular) function. It is not affected by water or protein intake and is, therefore, a more significant index of renal function than a measurement of blood urea.

(*c*) *Plasma potassium concentration.* Hypokalaemia warrants further examination for primary and secondary aldosteronism and Cushing's syndrome. It may be found, however, in connection with other causes, such as the abuse of laxatives or liquorice intake. Thiazide diuretics should not be given when the plasma potassium concentration is low. During long-term antihypertensive treatment that includes diuretics, plasma potassium concentration should be monitored. Hyperkalaemia may be a feature of advanced renal failure. Some caution is necessary when drawing blood samples, as forearm muscle contraction may elevate plasma potassium levels.

(*d*) *Electrocardiogram.* The ECG is used to detect signs of cardiac involvement caused by hypertension (left ventricular hypertrophy and strain, ischaemia and infarction) or of cardiac arrhythmias that may contraindicate certain forms of treatment. An electrocardiogram should be performed even in subjects with mild hypertension, as signs of slight left ventricular hypertrophy should be taken as an indication for beginning treatment.

The electrocardiographic diagnosis of left ventricular hypertrophy is rather difficult. It is customary to consider that the condition is present when the sum of the amplitude of the tallest R wave in leads V5 or V6 and that of the deepest S wave (in lead V1) exceeds 3.5 mV (the "Sokolow-Lyon" criteria). However, the limit of 3.5 mV is arbitrary, and a progressive increase of the index in serial electrocardiograms taken in the course of the disease is a clearer sign of developing hypertrophy.

Additional tests (optional)

(*a*) *Plasma sodium concentration.* The plasma sodium concentration is high in hyperaldosteronism, and may be excessively low in the hyponatraemic syndrome of malignant hypertension. (Plasma sodium is usually determined simultaneously with the plasma potassium concentration).

(*b*) *Fasting (or 2-hour postprandial) blood glucose.* Although this is an imperfect test for diabetes mellitus, its aim is to detect obvious additional cardiovascular and renal risks associated with hypertension. It should also help to identify the patients likely to develop diabetes mellitus with diuretic therapy. A glucose tolerance test may be performed to confirm a suspicious result.

(*c*) *Total plasma cholesterol concentration.* This is an important indicator of additional cardiovascular risk associated with hypertension.

(*d*) *Plasma triglycerides and HDL-cholesterol concentrations.* A plasma lipid profile obtained by measuring the fasting levels of triglycerides and high density lipoprotein (HDL)-cholesterol in addition to total cholesterol may predict cardiovascular disease better than the measurement of total cholesterol alone. Elevated triglyceride levels add a further degree of risk to an elevated plasma cholesterol. However, the risk of coronary heart disease is inversely proportional to the plasma level of HDL-cholesterol.

(*e*) *Plasma uric acid concentration.* Even though a high uric acid level is not, as such, a significant cardiovascular risk factor, it may influence the choice of therapy and may be affected by therapy (it is raised by thiazide diuretics).

(*f*) *Haemoglobin and haematocrit.* The anaemia associated with renal disease or other forms of anaemia may be detected. The presence of expanded or contracted plasma volumes may be detected in addition to abnormalities of haemoglobin concentration.

(*g*) *Urine culture.* May be useful in urinary infections.

(*h*) *Chest X-ray.* Information is obtained on cardiac size and contour, on the size and density (calcification) of the aorta, and on the presence of left ventricular failure. Rib-notching may be detected in coarctation of the aorta.

(*i*) *Echocardiography.* A reliable method for the assessment of left ventricular hypertrophy.

Extended evaluation

Complications of hypertension and suspected secondary hypertension may sometimes require special investigation. Because of their cost, poor return and, in some instances, risks and discomfort to the patient, these tests should be carried out only if indicated by the results of the initial clinical and basic laboratory evaluation. This extended evaluation is commonly performed by the hospital doctor or specialist.

(*a*) *Complicated hypertension*

(i) *Cerebral complications* may require one or more of the following investigations: electroencephalogram, computerized axial tomography (CAT), Doppler sonometry of neck and face arteries, and cerebral angiography.

(ii) *Cardiac complications* may be further assessed by echocardiography, coronary angiography, etc.

(iii) *Renal complications.* When further assessment of renal function is thought necessary, an intravenous pyelogram should be performed after checking for the few but sometimes serious contraindications (e.g., allergy, diabetic nephropathy). Renal function may be further explored by urine concentration tests, clearance measurements, urine culture, and renal angiography.

(*b*) *Secondary hypertension*

During the search for a curable cause of hypertension, one or more of the following investigations may be performed:

(i) *Primary hyperaldosteronism.* Measurement of plasma renin activity, plasma aldosterone concentration, and urinary aldosterone excretion may follow the finding of hypokalaemia. Low-renin and high-aldosterone levels are the hallmarks of the disease. The lesion may be localized by radiocholesterol scanning, adrenal venography, or CAT-scanning.

(ii) *Other adrenocortical hypertensions.* Measurement is made of plasma or urinary cortisol, its precursors, and metabolites.

(iii) *Renovascular hypertension.* After performing an intravenous pyelogram (or, alternatively, a radionephrogram), the lesion may be visualized by aortography or renal angiography. The functional importance of the lesion may be assessed by comparing plasma renin activity in blood sampled from both renal veins and by testing the response to the administration of antagonists or inhibitors of the renin–angiotensin system.

(iv) *Phaeochromocytoma.* Determination may be made of the 24-hour urinary excretion of catecholamines and their metabolites and plasma catecholamines (possibly noradrenaline, adrenaline, and dopamine separately). The tumour may be localized by aortography or an abdominal CAT-scan.

(v) *Aortic coarctation.* The lesion may be demonstrated by thoracic aortography.

A list summarizing the above laboratory investigations is presented in Table 7.

Table 7. Laboratory investigations

Strongly recommended tests
- Urine analysis
- Plasma creatinine
- Plasma potassium
- Electrocardiogram

Additional tests
- Plasma sodium (usually accompanies potassium determination)
- Fasting blood glucose
- Fasting serum cholesterol
- Fasting plasma triglycerides and HDL-cholesterol
- Plasma uric acid
- Haemoglobin and haematocrit
- Urine culture
- Chest X-ray
- Echocardiography

Extended evaluation (domain of the specialist)
- *Complicated hypertension*: tests of cerebral, cardiac, and renal function including intravenous pyelography.
- *Search for secondary hypertension*: measurement of renin, angiotensin, and aldosterone; corticosteroids; catecholamines; aortography and renal arteriography; adrenal ultrasound and computerized axial tomography (CAT); etc.

6
HOW TO DECIDE ON TREATMENT

WHEN the diagnosis of hypertension has been firmly established, the need for therapy should be considered. Except in rare emergencies it is not necessary to make a rapid decision; it is, on the contrary, far better to analyse thoroughly the diagnostic conclusion.

Any remediable cause that has been diagnosed, of course, should be taken care of without undue delay. If the patient is taking drugs or chemicals, such as hormonal contraceptives, liquorice or carbenoxolone, non-steroidal anti-inflammatory drugs, or corticosteroids, the practising physician should withdraw these substances. Patients with other causes should be referred to the respective specialist or to a hospital for further treatment.

If the diagnosis of *essential* hypertension is confirmed, the physician should evaluate the severity of the condition. In patients with severe (or moderately severe) hypertension the decision whether to treat will be taken without much hesitation. The methods of treatment are discussed in sections 7–10. However, most patients in whom hypertension is diagnosed for the first time have *mild hypertension*, and it is among this group of patients that it is difficult to decide whether to treat or not.

When to treat mild hypertension

Mild hypertension in adults can be defined simply as diastolic blood pressure (5th phase) readings *persistently* between 95 and 105 mmHg (12.7–14.0 kPa).[1] In practice, this means that non-pharmacological, general therapeutic measures should be started in a patient with mild

---

[1] Guidelines for the treatment of mild hypertension: Memorandum from a WHO/ISH meeting. *Bulletin of the World Health Organization*, **61**: 53–56 (1983).

hypertension and his blood pressure should be measured on repeated occasions over a period of 4 weeks. When the diastolic pressure falls below 100 mmHg (13.3 kPa) within 4 weeks, and remains so during repeated visits, further observations should be made over the next 3 months, and no drug treatment should be given; the general measures should be continued, however. In those patients whose diastolic pressure appears to be rising or is persistently above 100 mmHg (13.3 kPa) during the first 4 weeks, antihypertensive drug treatment should be started (Fig. 10 and 11).

For those who require continuing observation for 3 months, a decision to begin drug treatment should be made if, by the end of that period, the diastolic pressure still exceeds 95 mmHg (12.7 kPa). Patients whose diastolic pressure remains in the range of 90–94 mmHg (12.0–12.5 kPa), unless they require treatment because of high risk due to

Fig. 10. Definition, measurement, and management of elevated blood pressure

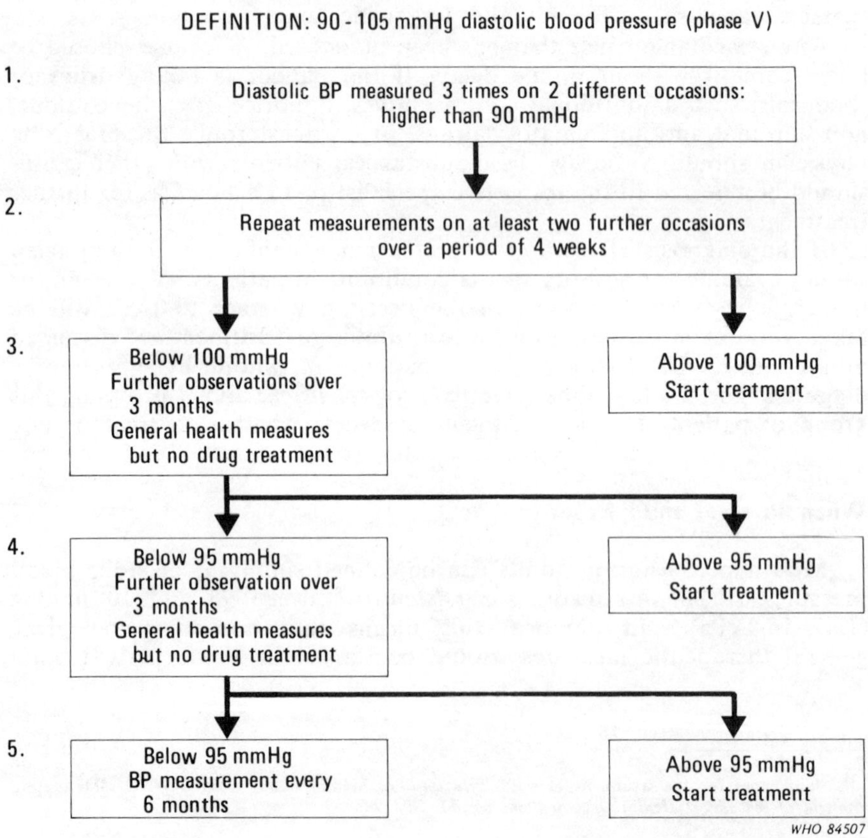

Fig. 11. How to proceed in mild hypertension

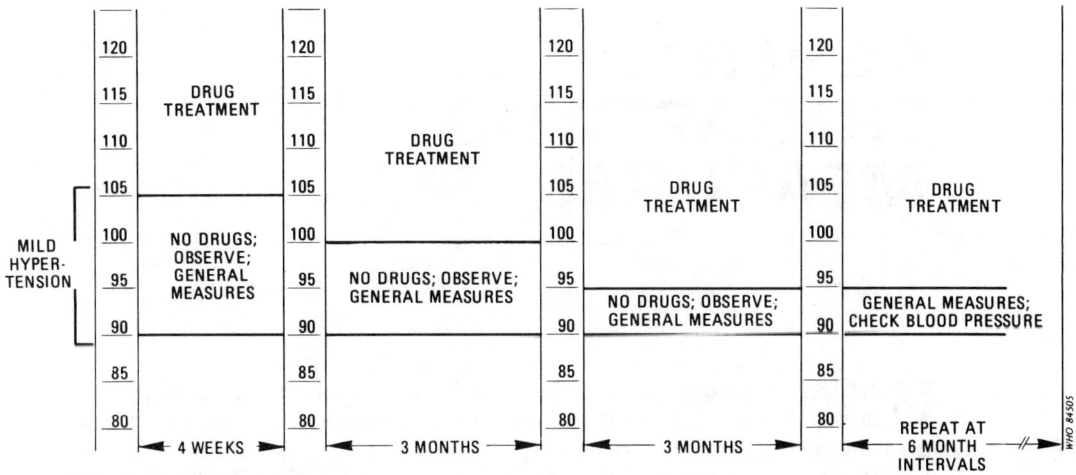

N.B. Only diastolic pressure is indicated on this scheme because therapeutic trials were based on these values; however, systolic pressure is equally important.

other associated cardiovascular risk factors, should be reassessed at intervals of about 6 months. If at any subsequent examination the diastolic pressure exceeds 95 mmHg (12.7 kPa) and remains above this level on repeated examinations, then drug treatment should be started. The treatment procedure for mild hypertension is summarized in Fig. 11, 12 and 13 (pages 47, 48).

Other factors influencing the decision to start drug treatment

Diastolic blood pressure is an important, but not the only, factor that influences the decision to begin drug treatment. The patient's need for drug treatment should be evaluated in a more comprehensive manner. Systolic pressure is at least as powerful an indicator of risk as is diastolic pressure.

Elderly patients (above 70 years) are less likely to derive long-term benefit from treatment and may experience side-effects with smaller doses of antihypertensive drugs (see section 9). If signs of involvement of the heart are present (left ventricular hypertrophy or coronary heart disease) drug treatment should be considered for even mild pressure elevations. If a patient has a *family history of stroke or heart disease*, drug treatment may be considered at lower levels. Finally, if a patient with mild hypertension suffers from an unassociated, potentially fatal disease, antihypertensive drug treatment is unlikely to affect the prognosis.

7 GENERAL THERAPEUTIC MEASURES

UNLIKE clinical drug trials with a double-blind design, the effectiveness of non-pharmacological measures in lowering blood pressure can hardly be demonstrated directly and with full scientific rigour. Many arguments in favour of the measures described below are based on clinical observations; some of these are of an anecdotal nature, others used "the patient as his own control" in alternating regimens. Further arguments in favour of these measures are based on pathophysiological considerations and reasoning, still others on epidemiological findings. However, unlike drug treatment, these general measures have no demonstrable harmful effects, except if grossly exaggerated. This is definitely an argument in favour of the general, non-pharmacological methods of treatment. They should be used to initiate any treatment of hypertension, and as continuing supportive therapy in combination with drug treatment.

Weight reduction

Although not all hypertensives are obese, many obese people do have elevated blood pressure. The first therapeutic measure in obese people should, therefore, consist of weight reduction, which in itself may result in a reduction in blood pressure. Weight reduction alone may correct mild elevations of blood pressure, while for moderate and severe hypertension in obese subjects, weight reduction and drug treatment should be combined. Weight reduction may be achieved by reducing the energy intake and increasing physical activity. Fenfluramine may be used as an adjuvant to weight regulation.

Salt-intake restriction

Reducing the intake of sodium chloride to below 400 mg (15 mmol) per day is consistently effective in reducing blood pressure, but, except for short periods, it is neither safe nor tolerable.

Controlled trials (albeit of only a few months' duration) in moderately severe essential hypertension have shown a small but worthwhile reduction of arterial pressure by modest, realistic sodium restriction (from 3.5 to 2.0 g, i.e., 160 to 90 mmol, per day), and also by potassium loading. However, similar studies in mild hypertension have not produced significant lowering of the blood pressure. The role of sodium restriction and/or potassium supplementation in the prevention of hypertension is under investigation.

Both weight reduction and salt intake restriction are behavioural interventions requiring a high level of cooperation between the patient and physician, and in many cases it may be quite difficult to achieve any therapeutic benefit. Although non-drug treatment of mild blood pressure elevation is preferable, in patients reluctant to adopt a low-energy intake and low-salt diet it might be more practical to commence drug treatment rather than to wait for a change in the patient's behaviour. However, the availability of antihypertensive drugs does not mean that the physician should not endeavour to obtain weight and salt intake reductions in his patient.

Exercise

Regular physical exercise may have a beneficial effect in subjects with mild hypertension though no trial has demonstrated a clear-cut change in blood pressure. However, the mental wellbeing, derived from regular exercise and the associated relaxation could be advantageous.

It has recently been claimed that exercise may prevent the development of atheroma by increasing the level of HDL-cholesterol but this has not been clearly established.

Individuals with moderate or more severe hypertension should avoid competitive sports, particularly if isometric exercise is involved.

Psychotherapy

The possible psychosomatic origin of essential hypertension has often been quoted as the rationale for treatment with yoga, acupuncture, transcendental meditation, relaxation, "autogenic training", musicotherapy, and other similar methods. While the efficacy of such methods has not been firmly established, they might be useful in selected cases to reinforce the patient's motivation to achieve useful behavioural changes.

Smoking and alcohol

Smoking, though not causally related to high blood pressure, is an important disease risk factor. Since the risk of coronary artery disease is some 50–60% higher in a hypertensive smoker than in a non-smoking hypertensive patient, vigorous antismoking advice should be given to any such patient.

The possible relationship between hypertension and alcohol intake requires further confirmation. There is some evidence that a slight alcohol intake may be of some benefit, perhaps by raising the HDL-cholesterol level and reducing atheroma.

Educating the patient

The success of both general measures of treatment and drug therapy depend on cooperation between the patient and his doctor or nurse. It cannot be overemphasized how important it is to explain to the patient the aims and purpose of antihypertensive therapy. This is especially true when, as in most instances, an apparently fit and symptomless person has to start drug treatment that will often be accompanied by at least some side-effects. The patient's wife, husband, or other family members should also be involved at an early stage in these discussions; the active cooperation of the family is invaluable in ensuring successful therapy. It is usually necessary to reinforce these explanations at frequent intervals during the first year of therapy and subsequently at less frequent, but still regular, intervals.

Small groups of hypertensive patients and their wives or husbands could be encouraged to have periodical discussions about their disease and related problems. These groups may be led by a physician or nurse, but the patients should be actively involved. The aim is to create an atmosphere of mutual support among the patients by using the psychological effects of group dynamics.

Physician and nurse should encourage rather than frighten the patient. Clearly, the way in which advice is given should vary with the patient's level of education and his personality. In general, advice should concentrate on the advantages of preventing long-term strain and damage to blood vessels rather than on more flamboyant references to the risks of death, heart attack, or stroke. In appropriate circumstances, the patient can be trained and encouraged to take his own blood pressure; this can be useful in encouraging compliance[1] as well as in assessing the effectiveness of treatment.

The patient needs practical advice on how to comply with suggestions for apparently simple measures that, in practice, involve very complicated changes of deeply ingrained habits. It is inadmissible to expect a patient to lose weight and follow a low-salt diet without explaining *how* he should accomplish this. In addition, the use of drugs should be explained at length and repeatedly, and the patient's comprehension should be checked on follow-up visits. In the past the

[1] Compliance: the disposition of a patient to follow medical or health advice.

patient has often been blamed because of poor compliance while, in fact, the real fault often lies with the health worker who has not acquired the skill of communicating with his patient, or does not have the time to give explanations that the patient can understand, or who does not care. Nurses may be more successful at educating the patient than doctors, since they are often psychologically closer to the patient and his family than a possibly paternalistic physician. The ideal patient education quartet is composed of the patient, husband or wife, the nurse, and the doctor, with each of the four members playing specific roles and being involved in multiple interactions.

Nurses may also be able to give better advice on weight reduction and low-salt cooking. It is beyond the scope of this manual to give details on reducing diets and low-salt cuisine, but some principles have to be stressed.

Weight reduction is a long and tedious process that can be best achieved by combining a moderate energy intake reduction and a simultaneous increase in physical activity. Amphetamine-like appetite-reducing drugs must be used with extreme care. Fenfluramine may be used as an adjuvant.

For *sodium reduction*, the health worker should be familiar with the sodium content of various foods (see Annex 2). The high-sodium and low-sodium high-potassium items can be identified at first glance. Sausages, cheese, preserved food, and bread are the main high-sodium foods of the usual, western-type daily diet – but, of course, the amount of sodium eventually ingested also depends on the salt added during cooking. Various types of table-salt replacement are commercially available; some of them include potassium salts that may be an additional asset for the hypertensive patient. From the culinary point of view it is important to compensate for the lack of taste of salt with other flavours, by using spices and other aromatic substances generously. Numerous cookery books dealing with this subject are available.

8
DRUG TREATMENT

DRUG therapy is desirable in the majority of patients with essential hypertension. It is also frequently necessary in secondary hypertension if surgical intervention is not possible or involves too great a risk, or in situations where blood pressure fails to return to normal values after the correction of an underlying cause.

During the past 30 years, continuous progress has been made in the development of antihypertensive drugs, and today it is possible to control the blood pressure of most patients who suffer from hypertension. However, apart from a few forms of secondary hypertension, treatment is symptomatic and empirical and not related to etiology for two reasons. Firstly, the causes are usually unknown and, secondly, the mechanisms by which several widely used antihypertensive agents lower the blood pressure remain unknown and open to speculation. It would be far better if the drugs could be chosen in relation to the cause and/or mechanisms of hypertension in a given patient.

How to lower blood pressure

Two important questions have to be answered: (*a*) how rapidly should pressure be lowered? and (*b*) how far should it be lowered? (i.e., should a complete return to normality be sought?). Except for the occasional hypertensive emergency it is neither necessary nor desirable to aim at a rapid reduction of blood pressure; a gradual reduction over several days, weeks, or even months is to be preferred. This is especially so in elderly patients, who are more sensitive to abrupt changes in pressure, and in those in whom a pressure, elevated for several years, has led to an adaptation of the circulatory system and to a resetting of the baroreceptor-mediated reflexes.

In principle, the ideal drug should reverse the haemodynamic changes characteristic of hypertension (increased total peripheral resistance and decreased cardiac output) and leave intact the baroreceptor reflex mechanisms. Pharmacological treatment of high blood pressure should aim to maintain the adaptive cardiovascular reactions to various stimuli and preserve circulatory homeostasis.

A stepped drug programme is recommended in order to achieve a gradual lowering of blood pressure (see page 46). Treatment should start with low doses of a single drug. The doses may then be gradually increased, but only with caution in the case of diuretics, since unwanted effects, mainly potassium loss, may be induced by increasing the dose. The daily dose of the diuretic should not exceed 25 mg of hydrochlorothiazide (or its equivalent). If adequate control cannot be achieved with full doses of a single drug, a combination of two or more drugs should be used.

In patients with advanced, chronic hypertension, it may prove impossible to achieve normal systolic and diastolic pressures, even with combinations of various synergistic drugs. In such cases, either reduced vascular compliance due to morphological changes of the arteriolar system prevents a sufficient reduction in total peripheral resistance, or the patient is unable to tolerate the diminution of pressure below a still elevated value. In such circumstances, however, one should still attempt to achieve a substantial reduction in pressure, even if normal values cannot be attained.

How to use antihypertensive drugs

Many antihypertensive drugs exist at present and their number is continuously increasing. The large number of commercially available drug combinations makes the choice even more difficult. In addition, the same or similar substances may be sold under different registered names in various countries. A recent textbook cites 135 such names of antihypertensive drugs—and it is not an exhaustive list.

Such an abundance of antihypertensive drugs may create considerable logistic difficulties and jeopardize adequate drug supplies in many countries. This applies not only to the treatment of hypertension but to other fields of pharmacotherapy as well. In response to this situation, WHO has established a list of essential drugs[1], which includes hydrochlorothiazide, propranolol, hydralazine, methyldopa, and reserpine. However, it is not possible to prepare a single drug list of general applicability because of the great differences between countries. Furthermore, in a fast-moving field such as the therapy of hypertension, any such list would be subject to frequent revision.

---

[1] WHO Technical Report Series, 1985 (in press) (*The use of essential drugs*: report of a WHO Expert Committee).

Table 8. Diuretics

Drugs	Site and mode of action	Side-effects and adverse reactions
hydrochlorothiazide or other thiazides bendroflumethiazide and chlortalidone, indapamide	inhibit sodium reabsorption in distal renal tubules	negative potassium balance, hyperuricaemia, hyperglycaemia, hypercholesterolaemia; reduced libido
furosemide and others	inhibit sodium reabsorption in the ascending limb of Henle's loop and in the distal tubules	pronounced diuresis, hypokalaemia, reduced intravascular volume, increased haematocrit, thrombosis
spironolactone	antagonizes aldosterone, excretion of sodium, retention of potassium	potassium retention (avoid in renal failure!), gynaecomastia
triamterene, amiloride	inhibit potassium excretion in the distal renal tubule, enhance slightly sodium excretion – only in combination with thiazide diuretics	potassium retention (avoid in renal failure!)

The various antihypertensive drugs may be classified, according to their mode of action, into the following four categories:

(1) Diuretics: drugs that enhance renal sodium and water excretion, and may secondarily reduce total peripheral resistance (Table 8).

(2) Drugs that act at various levels on the sympathetic system, including the alpha- and beta-adrenoreceptors (Table 9).

(3) Vasodilators, acting directly on the smooth-muscle cells of the arterioles, and calcium-antagonists or, more precisely, slow calcium-channel blockers (Table 10).

(4) Drugs that interfere with the renin – angiotensin system (Table 11).

Within the above categories, there are certain groups of drugs derived from the same substance or having similar chemical structures and only marginal differences in their effects. Groups, such as sulfonamide diuretics or beta-adrenoceptor blocking agents (beta-blockers) constitute drug families[1] and often will be referred to by such names. Individual drugs will be referred to by their generic names.

Since drugs regulate blood pressure in different ways, the combined use of drugs with different mechanisms and sites of action may result in a synergistic action, i.e., an enhanced effect will be achieved using small doses of each individual drug. Nevertheless, the aim is to reduce the

[1] Families of drugs: groups of chemically similar drugs with the same kind of therapeutic action.

Table 9. Drugs that act at various levels of the sympathetic system

Drugs	Site and mode of action	Side-effects and adverse reactions
adrenoceptor-blocking agents:		
propranolol and others	block $beta_1$- and $beta_2$-adrenoceptors	contraindications: bronchial asthma, heart-block greater than first degree, diabetes, bradycardia, peripheral arterial disease
atenolol, metoprolol and others	block $beta_1$-receptors more selectively than $beta_2$-receptors	
labetalol	blocks $alpha_1$-, $beta_1$-, and $beta_2$-receptors, (ratio alpha : beta, 1 : 4)	
prazosin	blocks $alpha_1$-adrenoceptors more selectively than $alpha_2$-adrenoceptors	postural hypotension (particularly with the first dose!) tolerance
reserpine	depletes noradrenaline stores in adrenergic neurons, reduces sympathetic tone	fatigue, drowsiness, depressive state, reduced sexual performance, parasympathetic dominance
methyldopa clonidine, and others	stimulates central alpha-adrenoceptors	fatigue, drowsiness, reduced sexual performance, reversible liver damage (methyldopa), bradycardia, rebound hypertension (clonidine), dry mouth (clonidine)
guanethidine and others	inhibits noradrenaline release, diminishes noradrenaline concentration in adrenergic neurons by inhibition of noradrenaline re-uptake	postural hypotension, diarrhoea, delayed ejaculation

blood pressure efficiently in the least complicated way, and therefore single drug treatment should be tried before combination therapy. There are, however, no rigid rules for prescribing and it may well be justifiable to begin treatment with a suitable drug combination, particularly if the dose of the individual components can be kept lower than in single drug treatment.

Some special comments on antihypertensive drug families

Diuretics. Among the numerous diuretics available, those that act on the loop of Henle (e.g., furosemide, bumetanide, or etacrynic acid)

Table 10. Vasodilators

Drugs	Site and mode of action	Side-effects and adverse reactions
hydralazine, dihydralazine	direct relaxation of arteriolar smooth muscle	flushing, headache, nausea, vomiting, tachycardia, angina, lupus erythematosus (high doses)
minoxidil	direct relaxation of arteriolar smooth muscle	tachycardia, fluid and salt retention
diazoxide (i.v.)[a]	direct relaxation of arteriolar smooth muscle	tachycardia, diabetes mellitus, pronounced fall of blood pressure
sodium nitroprusside (i.v.)[a]	direct relaxation of arteriolar smooth muscle (inhibition of chlorine transport)	high doses: danger of cyanide intoxication
calcium antagonists:		
verapamil	inhibit calcium entry into smooth muscle	bradycardia, a-v block, constipation
nifedipine	inhibit calcium entry into smooth muscle	tachycardia, headache, flushing, fall in plasma potassium level

[a] For emergency treatment only.

Table 11. Drugs that interfere with the renin-angiotensin system

Drugs	Site and mode of action	Side-effects and adverse reactions
captopril, enalapril	inhibit angiotensin-I-converting enzyme and consequently formation of angiotensin II	skin rash, disturbed sense of taste; high doses in patients with reduced renal function may induce proteinuria or granulocytopenia

are not suitable for the treatment of hypertension, except in renal or cardiac failure, because of their abrupt and drastic action. Thiazides and related compounds are generally more suitable because of their milder and prolonged action.

The combined use of two diuretics may be considered to be monotherapy, for example, the association of a thiazide with a potassium-retaining compound such as triamterene, amiloride, or spironolactone. The use of spironolactone is only indicated when aldosterone secretion is enhanced, as in primary or secondary aldosteronism. Triamterene or amiloride are only given together with a thiazide or a non-thiazide diuretic to maintain potassium balance. In general, however, the danger of hypokalaemia is low even during prolonged therapy, provided that the diuretics are given in low doses and the dietary intake of potassium is maintained at a suitable level.

Beta-blockers. All beta-blockers lower the blood pressure in a similar fashion and the choice of drug depends on individual tolerance rather than other factors. In comparison with the other drugs nadolol and atenolol act for longer. However, other beta-blockers compete by being prepared in special long-lasting, "slow-release" preparations. The contraindications, mainly asthma or bronchial constriction, are the same for the more cardio-selective beta-blockers as for those that bind to $beta_1$- and $beta_2$- receptors.

Calcium antagonists. Drugs, such as verapamil and nifedipine, that inhibit the slow-channel entry of calcium into vascular smooth-muscle cells have recently been recommended for antihypertensive treatment, either alone or in combination with a diuretic. Combination with a beta-blocker can be advantageous when nifedipine is used, as this will inhibit reflex tachycardia, but this combination should be avoided when verapamil is used as both drugs lower atrioventricular conduction. Verapamil and nifedipine have a relatively short duration of action, and delayed release preparations are available that are suitable for twice daily administration.

Inhibitors of the renin–angiotensin system. A new and promising development in the treatment of hypertension has been the discovery of inhibitors of the enzyme that converts the inactive decapeptide angiotension-I to the highly pressor octapeptide angiotension-II. Of the various inhibitors of the converting enzyme, wide clinical experience has been gained with captopril, which has been in routine clinical use for several years now; recently, considerable information has also become available from clinical trials with enalapril. Both compounds have been shown to be effective in lowering blood pressure, and even more effective when combined with a diuretic. Initial concern about some adverse renal and haematological effects of this class of compound (proteinuria, granulocytopenia) has been relieved by evidence that they occur only when large doses are given, especially in patients with renal insufficiency. Inhibition of the converting enzyme should also be avoided in patients with bilateral renal arterial disease. Safe and effective doses are: up to 150 mg of captopril per day (to be given in two doses); and 20–40 mg of enalapril per day (to be given in one or two doses). Skin rashes and disturbances of taste are occasionally reported, but they are reversible. Furthermore, with both compounds subjective disturbances have been reported to be quite rare.

How to select the drugs used

Various suggestions have been made on how to select the drug used to begin treatment. For diuretics and beta-blockers, various ideas have been proposed in an attempt to define a rationale for drug choice, instead of choosing the first drug by trial and error. For instance, it has been suggested that beta-blockers should be prescribed in younger patients and diuretics and calcium antagonists in the more elderly. However, apart from the difficulty in deciding where to draw the line between young and old, there are numerous other factors of greater significance than age when deciding on the drug of first choice. There are circumstances when contraindications or adverse reactions make a given class of drug unsuitable for monotherapy. Several years ago it was proposed that the selection of either a beta-blocker or a diuretic should be based on the level of plasma renin activity. However, many patients do not respond in the predicted fashion and the measurement of plasma renin activity cannot be justified in the vast majority of hypertensives. Thus, the choice depends upon the individual situation, the duration and the severity of the disease, the cardiovascular status, the presence of complications or of concomitant disorders, and, last but not least, on the personal experience and skill of the treating physician.

How to begin treatment: stepped-care programmes

Fig. 12 shows the stepped-care programme proposed in the report of a WHO Expert Committee on Arterial Hypertension in 1978. According to this scheme, treatment should begin with monotherapy using either a diuretic or a beta-blocker. In the light of experience accumulated since 1978, some additional recommendations can be given.

(1) All diuretics and beta-blockers should be started at relatively small doses.

(2) If, in beta-blocker monotherapy, the antihypertensive response to the initial dose is inadequate, the dose can often be increased after 2–4 weeks up to the maximum recommended dose for each compound.

(3) If the antihypertensive response to diuretic monotherapy is inadequate, recent experience suggests caution in increasing the diuretic dose beyond, for example, 25 mg of hydrochlorothiazide or chlortalidone per day, because of the risk of adverse metabolic effects.

(4) Wider clinical experience with converting enzyme inhibitors and with calcium antagonists suggests that antihypertensive therapy can now be started, with this type of drug as an additional choice to that of diuretics or beta-blockers, especially in view of the paucity of adverse subjective effects reported with some of the newer compounds.

(5) It is also possible to start treatment with drugs such as prazosin, labetalol, methyldopa, or clonidine, but care should be taken to begin

Fig. 12. A stepped therapeutic programme[a]

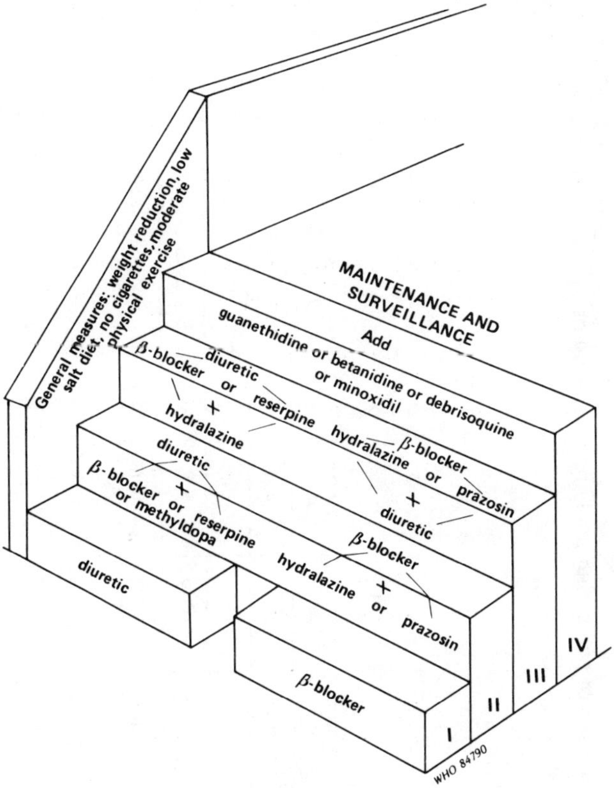

[a] Reproduced from: WHO Technical Report Series, No. 628, 1978 (*Arterial hypertension*: report of a WHO Expert Committee).

with small doses in order to avoid postural effects, especially with prazosin.

Combination therapy

If after several weeks or a few months of full-dose monotherapy, the blood pressure has not been sufficiently lowered, combination therapy should be started in preference to increasing the dose of the single drug (see Fig. 13). The aim of combination therapy is to achieve an enhanced effect with lower doses of two or more drugs acting at different sites.

A diuretic can be combined effectively with either a beta-blocker or a converting-enzyme inhibitor. A diuretic can be successfully combined

Fig. 13. Possibilities of combining antihypertensive drugs

	diuretic	beta-blocker	prazosin	reserpine	methyldopa	clonidine	hydralazine	minoxidil	guanethidine	captopril
beta-blocker	**yes**									
prazosin	**yes**	yes								
reserpine	**yes**	no	?							
methyldopa	**yes**	(yes)	yes	no						
clonidine	**yes**	no	no	no	no					
hydralazine	**yes**	yes	possible	**yes**	yes	yes				
minoxidil	must	must	?	possible	yes	yes	no			
guanethidine	**yes**	possible	no	no	(yes)	?	yes	yes		
captopril	yes	yes	yes	possible	possible	?	possible	possible	?	

▭ fixed-ratio combination available (not necessarily in all countries)

WHO 84506

with most of the other antyhypertensive agents, such as reserpine, methyldopa, clonidine, prazosin, labetalol, hydralazine, or calcium antagonists (both verapamil and nifedipine).

A beta-blocker may also be combined with an alpha$_1$-adrenoceptor blocker, such as prazosin, with a vasodilator, such as hydralazine, or a calcium antagonist, such as nifedipine. Care has to be taken when giving beta-blockers together with drugs that lengthen atrioventricular conduction time, such as verapamil, or others that cause a reduction in heart rate, such as clonidine, methyldopa, or reserpine.

The combination of a converting-enzyme inhibitor with a calcium antagonist has also been found useful.

The association of three or more drugs may be advantageous, if the response obtained with a two-drug combination is unsatisfactory or if the third drug helps to reduce some of the side-effects of the previous two-drug combination. One of the most widely used triple combinations comprises a diuretic, a beta-blocker, and a vasodilator, usually hydralazine. In this combination, nifedipine may be substituted for hydralazine. Instead of a beta-blocker, reserpine has also been used, but it has the disadvantage of causing unwanted central effects, especially sedation.

As a last resort, the powerful vasodilator, minoxidil (or guanethidine or one of the related substances, debrisoquine, betanidine) combined with a diuretic and a beta-blocker, may be tried, but the number of patients who need such complex combination therapy is small.

Free or fixed combinations

When two or more antihypertensive drugs are used, the question of whether the drugs should be administered separately or in a fixed-ratio combination has been widely debated. The advantage of giving the drugs separately is that the doses of each drug can be individually adjusted according to the response of the patient. However, the administration of fixed-ratio combinations facilitates treatment because the chosen ratio of the various drugs is generally selected on the basis of large-scale studies and will correspond to the needs of the majority of patients. It may be advisable to titrate the single drugs at the beginning of treatment, in order to find the optimum dosage and tolerance, and to switch later to the fixed-ratio combination that best corresponds to the dose of the various components previously administered separately.

The other advantage of fixed-ratio combinations is the small number of tablets that have to be taken, usually only one per day in many patients. It has been claimed that this improves patient compliance, which is so important in the long-term treatment of hypertension.

The use of fixed combinations is widespread in some countries, but severely criticized or even banned in others. For antihypertensive drugs, numerous valuable combinations exist and are accepted even in countries with very strict drug regulations. Because the aim is to obtain satisfactory control of blood pressure with one tablet daily whenever possible, the use of fixed combinations is inevitable in a large number of patients.

Adverse reactions and side-effects

None of the antihypertensive drugs is free of side-effects or adverse reactions, but it may be difficult to distinguish between unwanted drug effects and the unpleasant effects caused simply by the lowering of blood pressure. Long lists of side-effects exist, many of which have also been reported by patients in control groups taking placebos.

Reserpine, which reduces blood pressure by a peripheral mechanism but acts centrally as well, provokes drowsiness and, in addition, a depressive state, especially when given in doses above 0.5 mg daily.. Centrally-acting drugs, such as methyldopa and clonidine, cause drowsiness, fatigue, and reduce libido in male patients. However, fatigue, impotence, and nocturia may occur with various drugs and these effects increase with age. In most cases, subjective symptoms such as headache, nausea, flushing, drowsiness, and reduced alertness diminish with time and may disappear, often within weeks of starting the treatment. Postural hypotension is most pronounced with guanethidine and related drugs (betanidine, debrisoquine) while it may occur with prazosin as a first-dose effect.

Severe adverse reactions, such as systemic lupus erythematosus, have been reported after high doses of hydralazine, especially in slow acetylators. The syndrome is usually reversed after withdrawal of the drug. Impaired glucose tolerance may occur after prolonged administration of thiazide diuretics, which may also increase the serum lipoproteins and the serum concentration of uric acid. Indapamide has been reported not to induce undesirable effects on lipid or carbohydrate metabolism. The most serious metabolic effect of diuretics is hypokalaemia, which in a few cases may be severe and responsible for dangerous cardiac arrhythmias.

Failures

Failure to control blood pressure or escape from control poses the following questions:

(1) Does the choice of drug or drugs correspond to the needs of the patient? In particular, is the dose administered adequate?

(2) Does the patient take the prescribed drugs regularly?

(3) Is there secondary hypertension?

In all cases of hypertension the treating physician has a major responsibility to select the right drug(s), and to explain to the patient in detail the possible implications of the disease and its treatment.

The simpler the treatment schedule the more likely it is that the patient will comply with it. Although some recent studies have failed to show improved compliance with a once-a-day schedule than with two or three doses daily, the former regimen is to be preferred.

Self-measurement of blood pressure may encourage the patient to comply with treatment (see also section 2) and intelligent patients with moderate to severe hypertension may be taught to adjust their own treatment. Blood pressure records kept by the patient can also be used by the doctor in deciding on further treatment.

Treatment of hypertensive emergencies

Patients in whom a hypertensive crisis (left heart failure or epileptiform convulsions) has developed or appears imminent should be referred to hospital as an emergency, whenever possible.

Blood pressure in a hypertensive crisis has to be lowered, at least partially, by parenteral treatment. However, great care must be taken to avoid abrupt or profound drops in blood pressure beyond the limits of cerebral autoregulation. It may be sufficient to reduce the systolic blood pressure by 50–80 mmHg (6.7–10.6 kPa) and the diastolic pressure by 30–50 mmHg (4.0–6.7 kPa) depending on the absolute blood pressure values measured before the start of treatment. Thus it is necessary to produce a substantial reduction in blood pressure but not a rapid return to complete normality.

Various drugs are available for this type of treatment. Clonidine may be slowly injected intravenously or intramuscularly in a dose of 0.15 mg; if the effect is insufficient, 0.3 mg may be given 30 minutes later. Dihydralazine (hydralazine is not available in injectable form) may be given in doses of 6.25—12.5—(25) mg slowly, intravenously. Possible side-effects include tachycardia, headache, and angina. Labetalol may also be injected intravenously.

Diazoxide has been given in the past by rapid bolus injection, but slower infusion rates are now used, thus avoiding an initial precipitous fall in blood pressure. The dose used is 150 mg followed by 300 mg after 30 minutes if the response is insufficient. Sodium nitroprusside has to be given by intravenous infusion and blood pressure and heart rate have to be carefully monitored. The initial dose used in adults is 0.02 mg/min; this may be increased to a maximum of 0.9 mg/min. Long-term treatment with sodium nitroprusside should be avoided because of the danger of thiocyanate or cyanide intoxication.

Furosemide (40 mg given intravenously) should be used only if there is no dehydration. In patients with renal failure and fluid retention or pulmonary oedema, higher doses of furosemide may be indicated.

Nifedipine, in doses of 10 or 20 mg and administered sublingually, has been reported to be active in hypertensive crises. The same is true for captopril given orally at doses of 25–50 mg. With both drugs, blood pressure falls more slowly than after the intravenous administration of the drugs mentioned above.

* * *

Summary: Ten rules for the drug treatment of hypertension

(1) Blood pressure should be lowered gradually.

(2) Treatment should depend on the individual involved, according to the severity of the disease, the degree of haemodynamic disturbance, and other prevailing disease processes.

(3) Drugs should be prescribed in a stepped fashion starting with a single drug—except in cases of severe hypertension.

(4) Combination treatment is preferable to high-dose monotherapy because it involves the use of lower doses of the individual drugs and thus may cause fewer side-effects.

(5) Avoid giving inadequate doses of any drug.

(6) Never stop treatment abruptly or withdraw one drug suddenly.

(7) Familiarize yourself with a limited number of drugs and adhere to them. The newest drug is not necessarily the best one.

(8) Drugs that do not affect the mood and mind are preferable since they interfere the least with everyday activities.

(9) In most patients, treatment must be continued indefinitely. Do not change the treatment unless absolutely necessary. Treatment should be simple, if possible a single tablet a day.

(10) Have patience and train your patient to be patient.

9 HYPERTENSION IN SPECIAL GROUPS OF PATIENTS

Blood pressure in children

TO obtain accurate measurements of blood pressure in children, especially close attention must be paid to technique. Recommended cuff widths are given in Table 2 (page 12).

Special attention should be paid to checking the systolic pressure by palpation of the radial pulse when inflating and deflating the cuff. As already mentioned, in children the arterial sound may often persist until the cuff pressure has fallen to zero, and therefore, phase 4 is a better guide to the diastolic pressure. In children, as in adults, blood pressure should be measured in quiet surroundings in the absence of exciting or alarming stimuli, in a reassuring, friendly atmosphere (section 2).

Blood pressure in children depends on age even more than in adults (Fig. 14). The distribution of pressures is generally similar in boys and girls, both sexes showing a steep rise in systolic and, to a lesser extent, in diastolic pressure, between the ages of 5–15. The rise is correlated with sexual maturation. Children who gain weight rapidly are more likely to have a rapid rise in blood pressure as they grow up; therefore body size, as well as age, should be considered when evaluating the blood pressure of an individual child.

The definition of hypertension in childhood is at least as arbitrary as in the adult. Unlike in adults, little is known on the long-term prognostic value of blood pressure levels. This makes it even more difficult to delineate hypertension in childhood. However, children whose blood pressure is above the 95th centile merit special attention. It is likely that children whose blood pressure is relatively high are those who are likely to develop hypertension in adult life.

Apart from drug-induced hypertension, most forms of secondary hypertension are seen in childhood. Coarctation of the aorta should always be looked for in a child with elevated blood pressure.

Nearly all the wide variety of renal, adrenocortical and adreno-

Fig. 14. Percentiles of blood pressure (right arm, seated) in boys (left) and girls (right)[a]

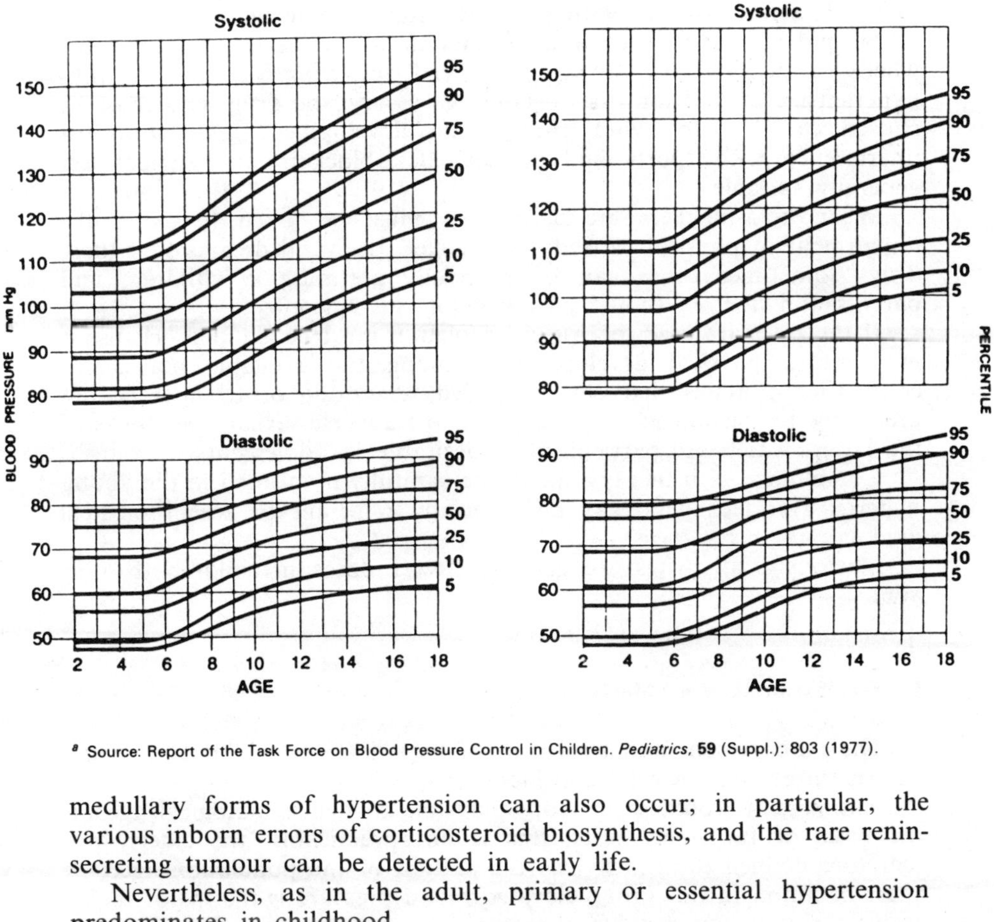

[a] Source: Report of the Task Force on Blood Pressure Control in Children. *Pediatrics*, **59** (Suppl.): 803 (1977).

medullary forms of hypertension can also occur; in particular, the various inborn errors of corticosteroid biosynthesis, and the rare renin-secreting tumour can be detected in early life.

Nevertheless, as in the adult, primary or essential hypertension predominates in childhood.

As in the adult, hypertension in children is usually without symptoms or signs, and therefore blood pressure should be measured whenever a child is being examined by the family physician or at school. Such routine checks provide valuable information, the child gets used to blood pressure measurement and this, in turn, lowers the risk of inducing neurosis.

There are, however, some characteristic signs that should alert the physician to the possible appearance of severe hypertension in a child. Failure to maintain the normal growth curve, and return of enuresis, for example, should always be an indication for blood pressure measurement.

Drug treatment is mandatory when the blood pressure exceeds the values at which treatment is started in adults. However, small doses of drugs may be given when the child's pressure is persistently 5–10 mmHg (0.7–1.3 kPa) above the 95th percentile for a given age.

Secondary hypertension in childhood should be dealt with surgically, whenever possible, to obviate the need for drug therapy. If antihypertensive medication does become necessary, the drug used must be chosen carefully to avoid growth and development retardation, or interference with sports and studies. Beta-blockers or thiazides are generally suitable.

When beta-blockers are used, care must be taken to avoid the impairment of physical capacity. Moreover, the vivid dreams that these drugs sometimes cause can be especially alarming in children, and parents and doctors should be aware of this side-effect.

If thiazides are used, potassium depletion must be avoided because it may retard physical development. Among the available potassium-conserving diuretics that can be added, amiloride or triamterene are preferable to spironolactone, because of the adverse sexual side-effects of the latter, which are particularly undesirable in adolescents.

Compliance with therapy should be carefully monitored in the young hypertensive; teenagers may be especially reluctant to accept medical guidance in this respect.

Obviously, all drugs are given at lower doses in children than in adults.

Hypertension in the elderly

The management and treatment of hypertension in elderly patients also requires some special considerations.

Although it would seem more plausible to define biological age on the basis of functional tests, this is not practicable; the elderly are therefore defined (arbitrarily) as the section of the population aged 70 years or more. In this group elevated blood pressure is the major factor associated with reduced life expectancy apart from age and sex.

However, to date no controlled trials have shown conclusively that by reducing high blood pressure the life-span of hypertensive patients above the age of 70 can be prolonged. In addition, no trials have been performed on patients with systolic blood pressure elevations alone. In elderly patients drugs more readily produce side-effects, both non-specific effects such as orthostatic hypotension, and specific effects related to a particular drug.

With the benefits of drug treatment largely unproven, extreme caution is needed when prescribing potent antihypertensive drugs for elderly patients. This is due to the fact that the pharmacokinetics of various drugs are often altered in the elderly. Diuretics are more liable to cause electrolyte disturbances, dehydration, disturbance of micturition, hyperuricaemia, potassium deficiency, and glucose intolerance. In the elderly, beta-blockers are more likley to provoke heart failure or conduction disorders such as atrioventricular block.

Some recommendations for the management of elderly hypertensive patients are listed below:

(1) The minimum number of laboratory and investigative procedures should be carried out. For example, intravenous pyelography should be performed only when drug treatment has failed to lower blood pressure, and even then only in those patients in whom surgery would be considered.

(2) Drug therapy should be given:

(*a*) to elderly patients with hypertensive retinal haemorrhages or exudates, hypertensive heart disease with left ventricular failure or congestive cardiac failure, cerebral or subarachnoid haemorrhage;

(*b*) to elderly hypertensive patients with symptoms that may be caused or aggravated by hypertension, such as angina pectoris, headache, or dyspnoea. Antihypertensive drug therapy will often be started if no other cause for these symptoms is found and continued if the specific symptom disappears and no side-effects are apparent.

(3) When drugs are used, the following rules should be followed:

(*a*) start with half of the usual adult starting dose;

(*b*) start with diuretics or beta-blockers (as in younger patients); the choice will often be determined by the presence of contraindications and of associated disorders that are frequent in this age-group. Thus, diuretics should be considered in the presence of congestive cardiac failure, and beta-blockers in the presence of angina and some tachyarrhythmias;

(*c*) centrally-acting drugs such as reserpine, methyldopa, and clonidine should be avoided because of the risks of depression, particularly disturbing in the elderly who are all too often prone to depression even without these drugs.

(4) Non-pharmacological measures have a more restricted role than in middle-aged subjects for the following reasons:

(*a*) weight reduction will be needed less often since obesity is less common in elderly hypertensives than in younger people;

(*b*) sodium restriction should be started gradually since reduced appetite may lead to a deterioration in general health;

(*c*) gentle, regular exercise should be encouraged more as a psychological measure to increase the quality of life;

(*d*) smoking is a common pleasure in the elderly. In this age-group the benefits of stopping smoking are undefined and may not justify that an elderly person be deprived of a lifelong habit.

Surgery in hypertensive patients

During anaesthesia and surgery, the blood pressure of hypertensive patients is more labile than in normotensive patients. Patients with a diastolic pressure greater than 110 mmHg (14.6 kPa) have an increased risk of cardiovascular complications in the perioperative period, and are particularly prone to myocardial ischaemia. Continuous ECG monitoring during surgery is therefore essential. Ischaemia is liable to occur during episodes of both hypertension or hypotension. Hypertensive spikes may be associated with laryngoscopy, or various surgical manipulations, and are liable to occur in the immediate postoperative period, even in patients adequately controlled with hypotensive drugs before surgey. Reductions of arterial pressure greater than 50%, or greater than 33% for 10 minutes should be prevented.

Elective surgery in patients with a diastolic pressure greater than 110 mmHg (14.6 kPa) is best deferred until the blood pressure has been controlled by appropriate hypotensive drugs: perioperative blood pressure control is improved by adequate preoperative treatment. Antihypertensive medication should be continued up to and including the day of the operation. Beta-blockers are generally safe and modify the pressor responses to intubation. Heart rate cannot, however, be used as a guide to hypovolaemia in such patients.

Anaesthesia impairs cardiovascular reflexes and as a result, arterial pressure during an operation is very sensitive to changes in blood volume. Hypotension is best treated with intravenous fluids while severe hypertension may be controlled by intravenous drugs such as sodium nitroprusside or labetalol. It is desirable to maintain the $PaCO_2$ (partial pressure of carbon dioxide) within normal limits during anaesthesia.

Patients with phaeochromocytoma present particular problems of management during operation. In these subjects, full alpha- and beta-adrenergic blockade should always be established before the operation and the anaesthetist should be prepared to give additional intravenous drugs during the operation if necessary. These drugs include the alpha-blocking agent phentolamine, the beta-blocking agent propranolol, and the combined alpha- and beta-adrenergic blocker, labetalol. There is no general agreement, however, on this point. Occasionally, hypertension during an operation has been difficult to control even with full alpha-adrenergic blockade; in these circumstances intravenous nitroprusside can be a most useful adjunct.

There is no convincing evidence that untreated patients with mild hypertension (diastolic pressure less than 110 mmHg [14.6 kPa]) are at increased risk from elective surgery. In patients with a higher arterial pressure, careful pre- and perioperative blood pressure control is essential.

10 THE MANAGEMENT OF HYPERTENSION IN PREGNANCY

AFTER the first trimester of pregnancy, peripheral vasodilation lowers the blood pressure below pre-pregnancy levels. For this reason, and because the affected population is young and fit, hypertension in pregnancy is diagnosed at the arbitrary limit of 140/90 mmHg (18.6/12.0 kPa); even lower limits may be appropriate for certain ethnic groups.

Pre-eclamptic hypertension

The commonest cause of hypertension in pregnancy is pre-eclampsia (pre-eclamptic toxaemia, toxaemia, pregnancy-induced or pregnancy-associated hypertension, or gestosis hypertension). This is a specific progressive disorder of the second half of pregnancy and can only be reversed by delivery. Pre-eclamptic hypertension is considered to be present when the systolic pressure is persistently at least 30 mmHg (4.0 kPa) and/or the diastolic pressure at least 20 mmHg (2.7 kPa) higher than the baseline levels from the first half of pregnancy.

The condition progresses in four stages (see Table 12). The pattern of evolution may differ with respect to its speed and time of onset; the two most difficult variants to deal with are rapidly progressive pre-eclampsia and early onset pre-eclampsia. Pre-eclampsia affects between 5% and 10% of all pregnant women and remains a major cause of maternal mortality, usually from cerebral haemorrhage. The perinatal problems (prematurity, intrauterine asphyxia, failure of intrauterine growth) are the result of placental ischaemia and infarction caused by obstructive lesions that appear in the uterine spiral arteries.

Relationship between chronic hypertension and pre-eclampsia

Chronic hypertension, that precedes and continues through pregnancy, is more rare and affects about 3% of pregnant women. Its

Table 12. Evolution of pre-eclampsia

(1) EARLY (1 week–3 months) –rising blood pressure –falling platelet count –rising plasma urate
(2) PROGRESSIVE (3 days–6 weeks) –controllable hypertension –proteinuria –reduced glomerular filtration rate –reduced fetal growth
(3) FULMINATING (6 hours–48 hours) –headache, abdominal pain, visual disturbances –uncontrollable hypertension –massive fluid retention –uraemia –disseminated intravascular coagulation
(4) TERMINATION –spontaneous labour –intrauterine death –eclampsia –abruptio placentae

obstetric significance is that it is associated with an approximately fivefold increase in the risk of developing pre-eclampsia. This explains the higher perinatal mortality observed in chronically hypertensive women; if they do not develop pre-eclampsia such individuals can expect a normal pregnancy.

General principles of management

There is no known effective medical treatment for pre-eclampsia; the condition can only be reversed by terminating the pregnancy with delivery. Patients with confirmed or suspected pre-eclampsia should be referred to a specialist without delay. Once established, pre-eclampsia is relentlessly progressive but remains asymptomatic until the terminal stages. Therefore management totally depends on adequate antenatal screening, early diagnosis, early admission to hospital, and a well-timed delivery.

Severe pre-eclamptic hypertension

Any patient with severe pre-eclamptic hypertension should be referred to hospital as *an emergency.*

The sudden increase in arterial pressure characteristic of pre-eclampsia is enough to explain the terminal cerebral pathology (eclamptic fits, haemorrhages). Therefore antihypertensive treatment is indicated if blood pressure recordings are 170/110 mmHg (22.6/14.6 kPa) or higher while the patient is at rest in hospital. Intravenous diazoxide in titrated doses of 30 mg per minute or intramuscular hydralazine at a dose of 10–20 mg, may be used in emergencies. Provided that excessive reductions in pressure are avoided the fetus is not compromised by this treatment. If the patient is symptomatic or convulsive, adequate anticonvulsant treatment should be given, usually either parenteral magnesium sulfate, intravenous diazepam or chlomethiazole. These measures are temporary expedients pending delivery.

Although excessive fluid retention is a feature of fulminating pre-eclampsia this is accompanied by a plasma volume depletion that will be exacerbated by the use of diuretics. Diuretics are, therefore, not administered unless the rare complication of left ventricular failure is diagnosed.

Conservative management of progressive pre-eclampsia is justified in the asymptomatic hospitalized patient before 32 weeks of gestation in order to enhance fetal maturity. In these circumstances blood pressure control is achieved by oral methyldopa (0.5–3.0 g per day) to which oral hydralazine may be added (50–200 mg per day).

Mild to moderate pre-eclampsia

Bed rest, restriction of weight gain, low-salt diet, diuretics, and non-specific sedation have all been advocated without any evidence of their efficacy. When pre-eclampsia has been diagnosed, the purpose of hospital admission is *not* to achieve bed-rest, but to provide day-to-day surveillance of an unpredictable, progressive, and dangerous disorder. It is known that the use of diuretics for the treatment of early pre-eclampsia is not beneficial and should be avoided. In general, no medical measure has been shown to retard or prevent the development of pre-eclampsia in its early stages.

Management of chronic hypertension in pregnancy

If maternal hypertension is severe enough to require treatment before pregnancy this is usually continued during pregnancy. There is, however, no evidence that the incidence of later, superimposed pre-eclampsia is influenced by the use of hypotensive drugs and the indications for their use thus remain strictly maternal. Treatment regimens may require modification to avoid unwanted drug effects on the fetus.

Effects of antihypertensive drugs on the fetus

Reserpine causes neonatal depression and is contraindicated. Methyldopa is the most widely-tested drug and does not appear to cause significant fetal or neonatal problems. Clonidine, betanidine, and debrisoquine have all been used but there is insufficient information available about any possible fetal side-effects to recommend their routine use.

Beta-blockers (including labetalol) have now been extensively tested in cases of pregnancy hypertension and seem to be safe. Captopril should be avoided.

11 CONTROL OF HYPERTENSION IN A POPULATION

THE control of any common disease requires action at the level of the population; each doctor may treat or even cure hundreds of individual patients, but the public health problem caused by the widespread disease may still remain. This is particularly apparent during epidemics of infectious diseases; for instance, an epidemic of malaria cannot be controlled in an area unless the swamps are drained or the mosquito habitats sprayed with insecticide.

For non-infectious mass diseases, the need for public health measures is less obvious; this applies especially to hypertension, because its causes remain mostly unknown. However, a number of general measures, for the population as a whole, and therefore beyond the reach of the individual physician, are virtually indispensable for the control of hypertension.

The prevention of hypertension

It is widely accepted that essential hypertension is largely a polygenic disease, but it is probably also environmentally conditioned as well. Obesity due to an excess energy intake and high sodium intake are the main exogenous factors, possibly leading to the development of hypertension in individuals with a hypertensive genetic background. However, the nutritional habits of a population, although usually deeply ingrained in a particular culture, are not impossible to alter. In fact, these habits are constantly changing as a result of developments in food technology, availability of nutrients, economic factors, publicity manipulations for commercial interests, and fashions.

In the same way, health-oriented changes in the nutritional habits of a population can be engineered by public measures, including regulations such as mandatory labelling of the sodium (and potassium) content of preserved food, commercial arrangements such as providing the market with low-sodium food articles, and—above all—by educating the public to prefer spices to salt and a lean body to a fat one.

It is likely, although as yet unproved, that the development of some of the new cases of hypertension in a population may be impeded or prevented by reducing salt intake and avoiding obesity. Since, in contrast to the administration of drugs for the prevention of disease in clinically healthy people, both measures are unlikely to harm the population, nutritional advice of this kind should become part of public health education programmes.

This type of education is known as *primary prevention*, to distinguish it from the prevention of the sequelae of hypertension by therapeutic measures, and should be started early in life. The best approach may be through school health education; this requires a good contact between health and education services.

Early diagnosis

Another aspect of hypertension requiring a public health approach is that, because the condition is symptomless, many individuals are unaware that their blood pressure is high. The need for the systematic detection of hypertension has been discussed in section 3. Whether done by mass-screening or by incidental screening (see page 16), this detection needs to be stimulated, even organized at the community level, in order to cover an entire population – clearly a task for the health authorities of a community, state, or nation.

Enhancing compliance by patient education

Subjects found to have hypertension should be followed up and treated by general measures and, if necessary, by drugs. The adherence of the patient to the prescribed regimens (his compliance) is often deficient, as shown by many studies. It can be improved, however, by patient-education programmes, by better organization of health services, by an active follow-up procedure, and by improved information and motivation of the practising physician.

Patient education may be carried out via the mass media, on a population- or nation-wide scale (television network or national press), but also at the level of the local community, through the local papers or radio station. The latter has the additional advantage that locally-adapted information may have a more direct appeal to the population of a smaller or medium-sized community such as a district or small town.

Counselling is another approach to the education of patient-groups (distinct from mass education). Groups of 6–12 patients, preferably with their partners, should meet periodically with the physician and/or nurse to discuss the questions related to their disease. Group dynamics develop under the guidance of the team leader (not necessarily the physician) and the psychological interactions created in this way enhance compliance with the therapeutic regimen, including the dietary changes. Such groups should be organized on a neighbourhood basis, and should be promoted throughout the community.

Improving the organization of health care

Deficiencies in the provision of care may considerably influence the compliance of a patient. For instance, an unpleasant, noisy, cold, untidy, or uncomfortable waiting-room may be the reason why patients miss follow-up visits to the physician. However, an attractive waiting-room with a friendly atmosphere may encourage the patient to return. The best solution is, of course, not to keep the patient waiting at all since any waiting is resented by the patient. It is recommended that the hypertensive patient (like any other chronic patient) be seen by appointment and that the timetable be adhered to. Medical practitioners may wish to consider seriously the introduction of a strict appointment system; it does not increase the workload, reduces the psychological tension of the patient as well as that of the physician and his/her assistants, and may greatly improve the compliance of the hypertensive patient. In social security or community- or state-owned institutions, it may be helpful to introduce appropriate regulations to begin an appointment system, if they are not already available.

An example of other organizational improvements that can be made is the introduction of a smooth referral system to be used when specialist advice is needed. However, as already mentioned, most cases of hypertension should be dealt with by the first-line physician. However, simple blood-pressure checks may be successfully delegated to appropriately trained nurses, and this may greatly improve the smoothness of the delivery of care to hypertensive patients. Finally, an adequate drug supply should be available to meet the requirements of the particular community.

Active follow-up

Whether treated by drugs or general measures, or if merely on observation, hypertensive patients should be followed up at regular intervals. If a patient misses an appointment, a reminder should be sent inviting him to come at another date. In the case of further non-communication, a health visitor or public health nurse should be sent to the patient's home to re-establish the contact. This kind of *active* follow-up is of great importance in preventing patients from dropping out of a therapeutic regimen and should be institutionalized, since the complications of hypertension occur much more often in "drop-outs" than in those who are under regular observation.

Whether hypertensive patients attend regularly is a question that can be easily monitored. Fig. 15 shows a file-card with a rider that should be moved at the end of each visit to the date of the next appointment. At any time a glance at the card-file (Fig. 16) will show which patients' visits are overdue. The card may also carry all the information on blood pressure, complementary investigations and treatment, and be used for easy morbidity reporting, if required.

Fig. 15. File-card with rider indicating next appointment

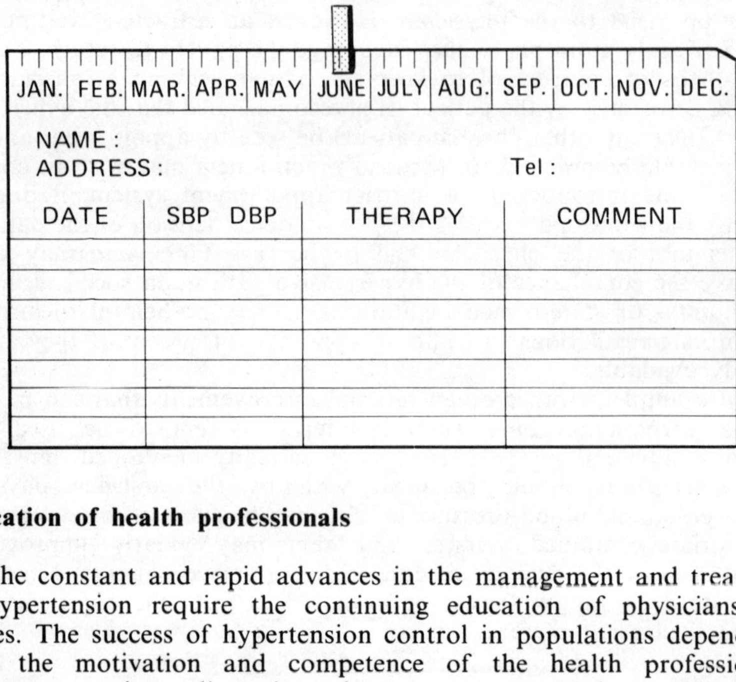

Education of health professionals

The constant and rapid advances in the management and treatment of hypertension require the continuing education of physicians and nurses. The success of hypertension control in populations depends on both the motivation and competence of the health professionals. Seminars, meetings, discussions, lectures, courses, update publications, etc., for physicians and nurses are therefore important components of the mass or community approach to the control of hypertension.

Hypertension control programmes

From the public health aspect, hypertension is a difficult problem and consequently its control in a population requires complicated action. Table 13 shows the 20 pivotal points of the control of essential

Fig. 16. Card-file by the end of May, showing 2 missed visits in March and April

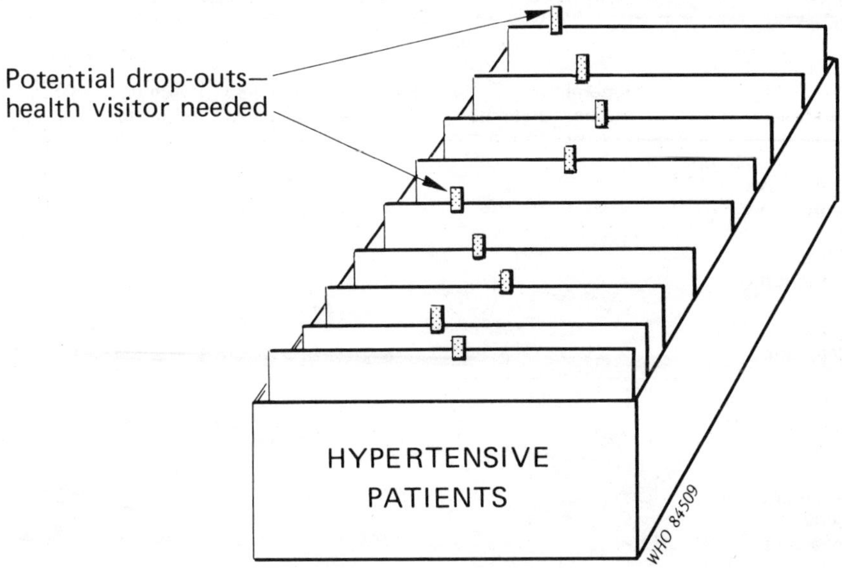

hypertension, all of which should be included in a coherent and coordinated programme.

Hypertension control programmes may be set up at international, national, regional, departmental, communal, or neighbourhood level. They may cover the general population of an area or defined occupational groups, such as factory workers. Those responsible for initiating and operating hypertension control programmes may be intergovernmental organizations, government health agencies, international or national scientific, lay, or mixed societies (such as heart associations or foundations and antihypertension leagues), and community health authorities.

Because of the particularly wide range of health problems associated with hypertension, control programmes should concentrate on hypertension, but at the same time they should form part of a comprehensive programme covering many other important aspects of health. Thus in a developing country with a limited number of health workers, a hypertension control programme should not drain the already scarce health manpower but should if possible employ medical assistants within the context of their usual activities. For example, where hormonal contraceptives are being dispensed in family planning clinics, a hypertension control programme should closely cooperate with those clinics and use them as a base for detecting hypertension. In countries where ischaemic heart disease is common, hypertension control should

Table 13: The 20 pivotal points of hypertension control in populations: all should be included in a control programme

Objectives	Education			Organization		
	General public	Patients	Health professionals	Improved services	Active follow-up	Drug supply
General population						
Salt-intake reduction	X		X			
Obesity reduction	X		X			
Early detection	X		X	X		
Hypertensive patients						
Adherence to follow-up		X	X	X	X	
Adherence to general measures		X	X	X	X	
Compliance with drug treatment		X	X	X	X	X

be part of a comprehensive project for the control of cardiovascular or chronic diseases. The optimum choice of a specific and/or comprehensive approach depends on the varied epidemiological, health care, and socioeconomic circumstances of a given population.

ANNEX 1

WHO PUBLICATIONS RELATED TO HYPERTENSION

1. WHO Technical Report Series, No. 168, 1959 (*Hypertension and coronary heart disease: classification and criteria for epidemiological studies.* First report of the Expert Committee on Cardiovascular Diseases and Hypertension).
2. WHO Technical Report Series, No. 231, 1962 (*Arterial hypertension and ischaemic heart disease: preventive aspects.* Report of an Expert Committee).
3. WHO Technical Report Series, No 628, 1978 (*Arterial hypertension.* Report of a WHO Expert Committee).
4. WHO Technical Report Series, No. 678, 1982 (*Prevention of coronary heart disease.* Report of a WHO Expert Committee).
5. WHO Technical Report Series, No. 686, 1983 (*Primary prevention of essential hypertension.* Report of a WHO Scientific Group).
6. WHO Technical Report Series, No 715, 1985 (*Blood pressure studies in children.* Report of a WHO Study Group).
7. WHO Technical Report Series (in press) (*Community prevention and control of cardiovascular diseases.* Report of WHO Expert Committee).

ANNEX 2

SODIUM AND POTASSIUM CONTENTS OF SELECTED FOODS[1]

	mg per 100 g of edible substance	
	Na	**K**
Fruit		
Apples, fresh	0.8	95.1
Apple juice	2	100
Avocado	3	340
Banana	1	420
Grapefruit	2	198
Grapes	2	250
Lemon juice, fresh	1	130
Melons	12	230
Olives, green, marinated	2400	55
Oranges	0.3	170
Peaches, fresh	0.5	160
Pears, fresh	2	129
Tangerines	2	110
Water-melon	0.3	100
Vegetables		
Beans, green, fresh	1.7	256
tinned	236	95
Beans, white	2	1310
Cabbage	13	227
Carrots	50	311
Cauliflower	16	400
Chick peas (dry)	26	797
Corn, fresh	0.4	300
Eggplant	0.9	190
Lentils, dry	36	810

[1] Based on: *Scientific tables*, 8th edition. J. R. Geigy, Basle, 1978, vol. 1.

	Na	K
Vegetables (*continued*)		
Lettuce, fresh	12	140
Peas, dry	42	880
Potatoes, fresh	3	410
Pumpkin	1	457
Sauerkraut	650	140
Soya beans, dry	4	1900
Sweet potatoes	5	530
Tomatoes, fresh	3	268
Cereals		
Cassava	4	20
Cornflour	1	120
Millet	3	430
Popcorn (unsalted)	3	240
Rice, boiled (unsalted)	2	38
Soya bean flour	—	1660
Wheat flour	2	290
Bread and pasta		
Noodles	7	157
Rolls	486	115
Rye bread	220	100
Spaghetti	5	22
White bread	385	132
Confectionery, sugar		
Chocolate, milk	86	420
Cocoa	60	900–3200
Marmalade	16	112
Sugar, refined	0.3	0.5
brown	24	230
Fats and oils		
Butter, unsalted	10	23
Coconut oil	0.4	0.4
Margarine	104	7
Pork-fat	0.3	0.2
Eggs, milk and milk products		
Cheeses:		
Melted cheese	1260	65
Soft cheese	606	74
White cheese, fresh	36	95
Condensed milk	112	314
Camel's milk	19	114

ANNEX 2 (*continued*)

	mg per 100 g of edible substance Na	K
Eggs, milk and milk products (*continued*)		
Cow's milk, fresh	55	139
Goat's milk	180	129
Hen's egg (per egg)	57	46
Ice cream	40	112
Milk powder	410	1330
Meat		
Beef, fillet	51	340
dried, salted	4300	200
Chicken	83	359
Corned beef	1300	60
Duck	85	285
Ham, smoked	2530	248
tinned	1150	293
Lamb	90	345
Pork, cutlet	62	326
Veal	90	330
Sausages		
Frankfurters	1100	230
Mortadella	668	207
Salami	1260	302
Fish and shellfish		
Carp	51	285
Eel, fresh	78	247
smoked	798	239
Herrings, marinated	1000	—
smoked	720	285
Mackerel	144	358
Shrimps	140	250
Sardines in oil, tinned	510	560
Trout	39	470

Note: As a rule, industrially processed food has high sodium concentrations (e.g., tinned juices; cheeses; biscuits, cereals, cornflakes; condiments and sauces such as mustard and ketchup; sausages, etc.) In food processed at home allowance should obviously be made for the salt added during its preparation, in addition to the natural sodium content of the ingredients. Beverages and mineral waters may have high sodium and potassium concentrations.

WHO publications may be obtained, direct or through booksellers, from:

ALGERIA: Entreprise nationale du Livre (ENAL), 3 bd Zirout Youcef, ALGIERS

ARGENTINA: Carlos Hirsch, SRL, Florida 165, Galerías Güemes, Escritorio 453/465, BUENOS AIRES

AUSTRALIA: Hunter Publications, 58A Gipps Street, COLLINGWOOD, VIC 3066 — Australian Government Publishing Service *(Mail order sales)*, P.O. Box 84, CANBERRA A.C.T. 2601; *or over the counter from:* Australian Government Publishing Service Booshops *at:* 70 Alinga Street, CANBERRA CITY A.C.T. 2600; 294 Adelaide Street, BRISBANE, Queensland 4000; 347 Swanston Street, MELBOURNE, VIC 3000; 309 Pitt Street, SYDNEY, N.S.W. 2000; Mt Newman House, 200 St. George's Terrace, PERTH, WA 6000; Industry House, 12 Pirie Street, ADELAIDE, SA 5000; 156–162 Macquarie Street, HOBART, TAS 7000 — R. Hill & Son Ltd., 608 St. Kilda Road, MELBOURNE, VIC 3004; Lawson House, 10–12 Clark Street, CROW'S NEST, NSW 2065

AUSTRIA: Gerold & Co., Graben 31, 1011 VIENNA 1

BAHRAIN: United Schools International, Arab Regional Office, P.O. Box 726, BAHRAIN

BANGLADESH: The WHO Programme Coordinator, G.P.O Box 250, DHAKA 5

BELGIUM: *For books:* Office International de Librairie s.a., avenue Marnix 30, 1050 BRUSSELS. *For periodicals and subscriptions:* Office International des Périodiques, avenue Marnix 30, 1050 BRUSSELS — *Subscriptions to World Health only:* Jean de Lannoy, 202 avenue du Roi, 1060 BRUSSELS

BHUTAN: *see* India, WHO Regional Office

BOTSWANA: Botsalo Books (Pty) Ltd., P.O. Box 1532, GABORONE

BRAZIL: Biblioteca Regional de Medicina OMS/OPS, Unidade de Venda de Publicações, Caixa Postal 20.381, Vila Clementino, 04023 SÃO PAULO, S.P.

BURMA: *see* India, WHO Regional Office

CANADA: Canadian Public Health Association, 1335 Carling Avenue, Suite 210, OTTAWA, Ont. K1Z 8N8. (Tel: (613) 725–3769. Telex: 21–053–3841)

CHINA: China National Publications Import & Export Corporation, P.O. Box 88, BEIJING (PEKING)

CYPRUS: "MAM", P.O. Box 1722, NICOSIA

CZECHOSLOVAKIA: Artia, Ve Smeckach 30, 111 27 PRAGUE 1

DEMOCRATIC PEOPLE'S REPUBLIC OF KOREA: *see* India, WHO Regional Office

DENMARK: Munksgaard Export and Subscription Service, Nørre Søgade 35, 1370 COPENHAGEN K (Tel: + 45 1 12 85 70)

ECUADOR: Librería Científica S.A., P.O. Box 362, Luque 223, GUAYAQUIL

EGYPT: Osiris Office for Books and Reviews, 50 Kasr El Nil Street, CAIRO

FIJI: The WHO Programme Coordinator, P.O. Box 113, SUVA

FINLAND: Akateeminen Kirjakauppa, Keskuskatu 2, 00101 HELSINKI 10

FRANCE: Librairie Arnette, 2 rue Casimir-Delavigne, 75006 PARIS

GABON: Librairie Universitaire du Gabon, B.P. 3881, LIBREVILLE

GERMAN DEMOCRATIC REPUBLIC: Buchhaus Leipzig, Postfach 140, 701 LEIPZIG

GERMANY FEDERAL REPUBLIC OF: Govi-Verlag GmbH, Ginnheimerstrasse 20, Postfach 5360, 6236 ESCHBORN — W. E. Saarbach GmbH, Tradis Diffusion, Neue Eiler Strasse 50, Postfach 900369, 5000 COLOGNE 1 — Buchhandlung Alexander Horn, Friedrichstrasse 39, Postfach 3340, 6200 WIESBADEN

GHANA: Fides Enterprises, P.O. Box 1628, ACCRA

GREECE: G.C. Eleftheroudakis S.A., Librairie internationale, rue Nikis 4, ATHENS (T. 126)

HAITI: Max Bouchereau, Librairie "A la Caravelle", Boîte postale 111-B, P-PRINCE

HONG KONG: Hong Kong Government Information Services, Beaconsfield House, 6th Floor, Queen's Road, Central, VICTORIA

HUNGARY: Kultura, P.O.B. 149, BUDAPEST 62 — Akadémiai Könyvesbolt, Váci utca 22, BUDAPEST V

ICELAND: Snaebjørn Jonsson & Co., P.O. Box 1131, Hafnarstraeti 9, REYKJAVIK

INDIA: WHO Regional Office for South-East Asia, World Health House, Indraprastha Estate, Mahatma Gandhi Road, NEW DELHI 110002

INDONESIA: P.T. Kalman Media Pusaka, Pusat Perdagangan Senen, Block 1, 4th Floor, P.O. Box 3433/Jkt, JAKARTA

IRAN (ISLAMIC REPUBLIC OF): Iran University Press, 85 Park Avenue, P.O. Box 54/551, TEHERAN

IRAQ: Ministry of Information, National House for Publishing, Distributing and Advertising, BAGHDAD

IRELAND: TDC Publishers, 12 North Frederick Street, DUBLIN 1 (Tel: 744835–749677)

ISRAEL: Heiliger & Co., 3 Nathan Strauss Street, JERUSALEM 94227

ITALY: Edizioni Minerva Medica, Corso Bramante 83–85, 10126 TURIN; Via Lamarmora 3, 20100 MILAN

JAPAN: Maruzen Co. Ltd., P.O. Box 5050, TOKYO International, 100–31

JORDAN: Jordan Book Centre Co. Ltd., University Street, P.O. Box 301 (Al-Jubeiha), AMMAN

KUWAIT: The Kuwait Bookshops Co. Ltd., Thunayan Al-Ghanem Bldg, P.O. Box 2942, KUWAIT

LAOS PEOPLE'S DEMOCRATIC REPUBLIC: The WHO Programme Coordinator, P.O. Box 343, VIENTIANE

LEBANON: The Levant Distributors Co. S.A.R.L., Box 1181, Makdassi Street, Hanna Bldg, BEIRUT

LUXEMBOURG: Librairie du Centre, 49 bd Royal, LUXEMBOURG

MALAWI: Malawi Book Service, P.O. Box 30044, Chichiti, BLANTYRE 3

WHO publications may be obtained, direct or through booksellers, from:

MALAYSIA: The WHO Programme Coordinator, Room 1004, 10th Floor, Wisma Lim Foo Yong (formerly Fitzpatrick's Building), Jalan Raja Chulan, KUALA LUMPUR 05–10; P.O. Box 2550, KUALA LUMPUR 01–02; Parry's Book Center, K.L. Hilton Hotel, Jln. Treacher, P.O. Box 960, KUALA LUMPUR

MALDIVES: *See* India, WHO Regional Office

MEXICO: Libreria Internacional, S.A. de C.V., Av. Sonora 206, 06100-MÉXICO, D.F.

MONGOLIA: *see* India, WHO Regional Office

MOROCCO: Editions La Porte, 281 avenue Mohammed V, RABAT

MOZAMBIQUE: INLD, Caixa Postal 4030, MAPUTO

NEPAL: *see* India, WHO Regional Office

NETHERLANDS: Medical Books Europe BV, Noorderwal 38, 7241 BL LOCHEM

NEW ZEALAND: Government Printing Office, Publications Section, Mulgrave Street, Private Bag, WELLINGTON 1; Walter Street, WELLINGTON; World Trade Building, Cubacade, Cuba Street, WELLINGTON. *Government Bookshops at:* Hannaford Burton Building, Rutland Street, Private Bag, AUCKLAND; 159 Hereford Street, Private Bag, CHRISTCHURCH; Alexandra Street, P.O. Box 857, HAMILTON; T & G Building, Princes Street, P.O. Box 1104, DUNEDIN — R. Hill & Son Ltd, Ideal House, Cnr Gillies Avenue & Eden Street, Newmarket, AUCKLAND 1

NIGERIA: University Bookshop Nigeria Ltd, University of Ibadan, IBADAN

NORWAY: J. G. Tanum A/S, P.O. Box 1177 Sentrum, OSLO 1

PAKISTAN: Mirza Book Agency, 65 Shahrah–E–Quaid–E–Azam, P.O. Box 729, LAHORE 3; Sasi Limited, Sasi Centre, G.P.O. Box 779, I.I. Chundrigar Road, KARACHI

PAPUA NEW GUINEA: The WHO Programme Coordinator, P.O. Box 646, KONEDOBU

PHILIPPINES: World Health Organization, Regional Office for the Western Pacific, P.O. Box 2932, MANILA — The Modern Book Company Inc., P.O. Box 632, 922 Rizal Avenue, MANILA 2800

POLAND: Składnica Ksiegarska, ul Mazowiecka 9, 00052 WARSAW *(except periodicals)* — BKWZ Ruch, ul Wronia 23, 00840 WARSAW *(periodicals only)*

PORTUGAL: Livraria Rodrigues, 186 Rua do Ouro, LISBON 2

REPUBLIC OF KOREA: The WHO Programme Coordinator, Central P.O. Box 540, SEOUL

SIERRA LEONE: Njala University College Bookshop (University of Sierra Leone), Private Mail Bag, FREETOWN

SINGAPORE: The WHO Programme Coordinator, 144 Moulmein Road, SINGAPORE 1130; Newton P.O. Box 31, SINGAPORE 9122 — Select Books (Pte) Ltd, Tanglin Shopping Centre, 19 Tanglin Road 03–15, SINGAPORE 10

SOUTH AFRICA: *Contact major book stores*

SPAIN: Ministerio de Sanidad y Consumo, Servicio de Publicaciones, Paseo del Prado 18–20, MADRID–14 — Comercial Atheneum S.A., Consejo de Ciento 130–136, 08015 BARCELONA; General Moscardó 29, MADRID 20 — Libreria Díaz de Santoz, Lagasca 95 y Maldonado 6, MADRID 6; Balmes 417 y 419, 08022 BARCELONA

SRI LANKA: *see* India, WHO Regional Office

SWEDEN: *For books:* Aktiebolaget C.E. Fritzes Kungl. Hovbokhandel, Regeringsgatan 12, 103 27 STOCKHOLM. *For periodicals:* Wennergren-Williams AB, Box 30004, 104 25 STOCKHOLM

SWITZERLAND: Medizinischer Verlag Hans Huber, Länggass Strasse 76, 3012 BERNE 9

THAILAND: *see* India, WHO Regional Office

TUNISIA: Société Tunisienne de Diffusion, 5 avenue de Carthage, TUNIS

TURKEY: Haset Kitapevi, 469 Istiklal Caddesi, Beyoglu, ISTANBUL

UNITED KINGDOM: H.M. Stationery Office: 49 High Holborn, LONDON WC1V 6HB; 13a Castle Street, EDINBURGH EH2 3AR, 80 Chichester Street, BELFAST BT1 4JY; Brazennose Street, MANCHESTER M60 8AS; 258 Broad Street, BIRMINGHAM B1 2HE; Southey House, Wine Street, BRISTOL BS1 2BQ. *All mail orders should be sent to:* HMSO Publications Centre, 51 Nine Elms Lane, LONDON SW8 5DR

UNITED STATES OF AMERICA: *Copies of individual publications (not subscriptions):* WHO Publications Center USA, 49 Sheridan Avenue, ALBANY, NY 12210. *Subscription orders and correspondence concerning subscriptions should be addressed to the* World Health Organization, Distribution and Sales, 1211 GENEVA 27, Switzerland. *Publications are also available from the* United Nations Bookshop, NEW YORK, NY 10017 (*retail only*)

URUGUAY: Libreria Agropecuaria S.R.L., Casilla de Correo 1755, Alzaibar 1328, MONTEVIDEO

USSR: *For readers in the USSR requiring Russian editions:* Komsomolskij prospekt 18, Medicinskaja Kniga, MOSCOW — *For readers outside the USSR requiring Russian editions:* Kuzneckij most 18, Meždunarodnaja Kniga, MOSCOW G-200

VENEZUELA: Libreria del Este, Apartado 60.337, CARACAS 106 — Libreria Medica Paris, Apartado 60.681, CARACAS 106

YUGOSLAVIA: Jugoslovenska Knjiga, Terazije 27/II, 11000 BELGRADE

ZAIRE: Librairie universitaire, avenue de la Paix Nº 167, B.P. 1682, KINSHASA I

Special terms for developing countries are obtainable on application to the WHO Programme Coordinators or WHO Regional Offices listed above or to the World Health Organization, Distribution and Sales Service, 1211 Geneva 27, Switzerland. Orders from countries where sales agents have not yet been appointed may also be sent to the Geneva address, but must be paid for in pounds sterling, US dollars, or Swiss francs. Unesco book coupons may also be used.

Prices are subject to change without notice.